Foot Health Training Guide
for Long-Term Care Personnel

D1256829

Foot Health Training Guide for Long-Term Care Personnel

by
Arthur E. Helfand, D.P.M.
Professor Emeritus

with selected contributions by
Albert J. Finestone, M.D., M.Sc.
Adjunct Professor of Medicine

and
Roberta A. Newton, P.T., Ph.D.
Professor of Physical Therapy and Medicine

Temple University, School of Podiatric Medicine,
School of Medicine, and College of Allied Health Professions

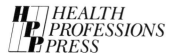
HEALTH
PROFESSIONS
PRESS

Baltimore • London • Sydney

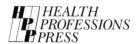
HEALTH
PROFESSIONS
PRESS

Health Professions Press, Inc.
Post Office Box 10624
Baltimore, Maryland 21285-0624

www.healthpropress.com

Typeset by Integrated Publishing Solutions, Grand Rapids, Michigan.
Manufactured in the United States of America by
Versa Press, Inc., East Peoria, Illinois.

All of the photographs in this book were provided by Arthur E. Helfand, D.P.M.

The publisher and the author have made every effort to ensure that all of the
information and instructions given in this book are accurate and safe, but they
cannot accept liability for any resulting injury, damage, or loss to either person
or property, whether direct or consequential and however it occurs. Medical
care and/or advice should only be provided under the direction of a licensed
health care professional.

Library of Congress Cataloging-in-Publication Data

Helfand, Arthur E.
   Foot health training guide for long-term care personnel / by Arthur E. Helfand ;
with selected contributions by Albert J. Finestone and Roberta A. Newton.
     p.   cm.
   Includes bibliographical references and index.
   ISBN-13: 978-1-932529-32-6 (pbk.)
   ISBN-10: 1-932529-32-2 (pbk.)
   1. Older people—Long-term care.   2. Feet—Care and hygiene.   I. Finestone,
Albert J.   II. Newton, Roberta A.   III. Title.
   [DNLM: 1. Foot Diseases—diagnosis.   2. Foot Diseases—prevention & control.
3. Long-Term Care—methods.   WE 880 H4736f 2007]
RA564.8.F664 2007
610.73'6—dc22   2006025685

British Library Cataloguing in Publication data are available from the
British Library.

Contents

About the Author

Arthur E. Helfand, D.P.M., graduated from Temple University in Philadelphia with a doctor of podiatric medicine degree in 1957 and completed his residency training at St. Luke's Hospital and Children's Medical Center in Philadelphia. Currently Professor Emeritus at Temple University's School of Podiatric Medicine, Dr. Helfand is also Adjunct Professor of Medicine at Temple University School of Medicine; a member of the honorary staff at Temple University Hospital and Thomas Jefferson University Hospital; a consultant to Temple University's Institute on Aging; and retired Professor and Chair of the Department of Community Health, Aging, and Health Policy at Temple University, School of Podiatric Medicine. Dr. Helfand practiced clinically for 45 years in Philadelphia.

Dr. Helfand is Fellow, The College of Physicians of Philadelphia. In addition, he is a member of the Task Force on Aging of the American Public Health Association, a member of the Board of Directors of the Philadelphia Corporation for Aging, and a member of the Stakeholders Group on Diabetes for the Pennsylvania Department of Health. He has authored or co-authored 337 papers, teaching programs, and book chapters and has edited 6 textbooks dealing with podogeriatrics, rehabilitation of the foot, and podiatric public health.

About the Contributors

Albert J. Finestone, M.D., M.Sc., is board certified in internal medicine and geriatrics and has practiced in both fields for many years. At Temple University's School of Medicine, he is Director of the Institute on Aging; Adjunct Professor of Medicine; and Associate Dean, Emeritus, for the Office of Continuing Medical Education (CME). During his tenure as Associate Dean for CME, his major objective was to change physician behavior to best practice.

Dr. Finestone is Fellow, The College of Physicians of Philadelphia. He is also Project Director of the Geriatric Education Center of Pennsylvania, a consortium among the University of Pittsburgh, The Pennsylvania State University, and Temple University. He has authored 100 papers, books, and book chapters.

Roberta A. Newton, P.T., Ph.D., is Professor of Physical Therapy, Professor of Medicine, and Associate Director of Temple University's Institute on Aging. She received her doctoral degree in neurophysiology at the Medical College of Virginia. For more than 30 years, she taught and conducted research at the Medical College of Virginia and Temple University.

Dr. Newton is Fellow, The College of Physicians of Philadelphia and the Gerontological Society of America. Her education, research, and service focus is directed toward balance control and predictors of falls in older adults and toward the development of effective fall reduction programs (see http://www.temple.edu/older_adult). She developed and validated the Multi-Directional Reach Test (MDRT) as a measure of balance stability in community-dwelling older adults and in older adults who have a history of falling. She is an internationally recognized expert in the area of falls and fall prevention programming, as evidenced by her publications, national and international presentations, and funding records.

Foreword

It has been established that the maintenance of independence is a key to a longer life. However, some older adults for various reasons lose some degree of independence when they transfer to long-term care (LTC). Once in a LTC facility, the ability to walk is a very important factor in the quality of life. Dr. Arthur E. Helfand, the author of *Foot Health Training Guide for Long-Term Care Personnel,* has produced a valuable resource for helping LTC staff support the mobility and quality of life of residents. Dr. Helfand is a distinguished expert in podiatric medicine, and his book clearly covers all issues involved in podogeriatrics.

I am a general internist and a geriatrician; in my many years of practice and observing other physicians, I have noted that the mouth and the feet are two areas of the human body that are poorly examined by physicians and other health professionals. I believe that professionals in LTC facilities would significantly improve their ability to help older residents by reading this book. However, this group of professionals in LTC facilities must pay attention to all of the other areas that would have an impact on these individuals in terms of foot care. First, many of these residents have some degree of dementia and are unable to communicate clearly with the LTC staff. Second, visual and hearing problems are very common, so communications between professionals and residents are impaired. The impact of medications on cognition also must be considered. Many of these individuals have problems with depression, dizziness and vertigo, pain, nutritional problems, gastrointestinal problems, neurological problems, and degenerative joint disease. In addition, they may have chronic heart failure, renal disease, and nutritional problems, which can cause lower extremity edema and obscure some of the podiatric problems. Finally, many of these individuals may have diabetes, which can produce neurological and circulatory problems. Therefore, LTC professionals must recognize that these individuals can have significant problems with their feet and have no complaints. Pressure areas as well as circulatory problems in the lower extremities must be evaluated carefully.

My final message to the reader is that the history and the physical examination are important, but in these individuals, careful observation is the key to good care and may help prevent serious complications in the lower extremities. Diabetes and spinal stenosis impair pain sensation in the lower extremities, so physical examination of the lower extremities becomes increasingly important.

In summary, the feet, as part of the human body, are affected by normal aging, disease, drugs, environment, and so forth, so all of the factors must be considered. Dr. Helfand's book raises the awareness and understanding of care staff regarding all of these issues and will contribute to high-quality foot care in LTC facilities.

Albert J. Finestone, M.D., M.Sc.
Professor of Medicine
Temple University, School of Medicine
Associate Dean CME, Emeritus
Consortium Project Director, Geriatric Education Center of Pennsylvania
Director, Temple University, Institute on Aging

Preface

The inclusion of appropriate podiatric services in long-term care programs often will produce dramatic effects. Immobility can be replaced by activity. Quality of care translates into quality of life. Support and encouragement can be directed to independence and a strong sense of personal identity and worth. Isolation can be replaced by interaction. When the quality of life decreases as a result of disease, disability, or age, those precious aspects of dignity must be restored to a maximum level by caring staff and people. Because mobility is an important catalyst for life, podiatric care can help to restore some of the lost dignity by keeping residents walking and moving about so that they can accept and participate in the social activities that are provided by the facility.

One of the health goals of the United States is to upgrade the quality of care that is offered by nursing and long-term care facilities so that older residents and patients with chronic diseases and disabilities can maintain a maximum quality of life. The purpose of this educational program guide is to sensitize staff members to recognize foot and related lower extremity conditions at their earliest manifestations; recognize the need for early consultation and management; use health promotion, prevention, and education; and adopt plans for continuing surveillance and care. This text is intended to serve as a short-term training program and a reference for future activities.

It has long been recognized that pedal health is necessary to independent activity, individual dignity, and the general well-being of long-term care residents. Problems that contribute to disability and pain commonly lead to inactivity, listlessness, and deterioration of mental as well as physical health. This guide is designed to share knowledge and skills and increase the awareness of long-term care personnel to foot and related health needs. It is my hope that residents, patients, and staff members will benefit by initiating early assessment and preventive and remedial interventions and measures to allow older individuals to live their lives as fully as possible to the end of life.

Acknowledgments

The preparation of this text has had a long evolutionary history. I had the privilege of being a part of each of these special programs. The initial concept to provide education for long-term care professionals was initiated at the University of Nebraska by a federally funded traineeship with the cooperative efforts of John R. Carson, M.A., Edward L. Tarara, D.P.M., and Marvin W. Shapiro, D.P.M. (deceased). The Commonwealth of Pennsylvania, through its Department of Aging—including Secretary Elias S. Cohen and Secretary Nora Dowd Eisenhower—recognized a need for foot health as an important component in geriatric care. The Pennsylvania Diabetes Academy; the Foundation for the Pennsylvania Medical Society; Kathleen M. Dwyer, R.D., Ph.D.; and the Pennsylvania Department of Health gave their support and special interest in foot care as it relates to older diabetic patients, as well as the funding to develop a comprehensive podogeriatric assessment protocol. The American Podiatric Medical Association, in cooperation with the U.S. Department of Health and Human Services, continued to recognize the need for foot health for older patients, especially in long-term care facilities. The U.S. Department of Veterans Affairs and retired Director of the Podiatric Service, Martin Mussman, D.P.M., ensured that podiatric care and training remained a part of long-term care. The Joint Commission on Accreditation of Health Care Organizations initiated foot health standards and training. Temple University—through its School of Podiatric Medicine and Institute on Aging and, in particular, through Albert J. Finestone, M.D., M.Sc.; Roberta A. Newton, Ph.D., P.T.; and the Geriatric Education Center of Pennsylvania—expanded the information on podogeriatric assessment and special educational programs. The University of Pennsylvania School of Nursing continued to include comprehensive podogeriatric assessment in its educational programs. The Board of Directors of the Eastern Pennsylvania Geriatrics Society supported interdisciplinary geriatric education.

I am deeply indebted for the assistance and encouragement given by my wife, Myra W. Helfand, who carried out the massive task of proofreading this text and making sure that language had mean-ing and who permitted me to take the time to prepare this book. And finally, the staff at Health Professions Press was supportive by recog-nizing a need to help older and long-term care patients live their lives with dignity and live life to the end of life.

To my wife,
Myra,
and our children,
Jennifer Bess and Lewis Aaron.
With all of my love.

Introduction

Geriatrics is the branch of medicine that treats the problems of aging. It is more restricted in scope than gerontology, the scientific study of the clinical, biological, historical, and sociological aspects of old age. Podogeriatrics is the special area of podiatric practice that refers to the treatment of foot problems that affect aging individuals. Medical treatment of older adults presents a challenge because many of them have numerous physical problems that complicate and interfere with the diagnosis and treatment of any single illness. Diseases of one organ system place stress on other systems; furthermore, some diseases do not produce in older adults the symptoms that usually are seen in younger individuals. Many older adults also have nutritional deficiencies because of limited incomes, poor oral health, and other problems. In addition, older adults have increased risks for complications from surgery, and convalescence takes longer because damaged tissues recover more slowly. The longer periods of bed rest also can lead to pneumonia, bedsores, and circulatory disorders. Drugs are metabolized more slowly as well, and their effects are prolonged in the body.

EPIDEMIOLOGY

Old age has increasingly significant political, medical, economic, social, and demographic consequences for all nations. Although the percentage of people who are 65 years and older now ranges from approximately 13% to 20% in industrialized countries, these percentages, or the actual numbers that they represent, are expected to increase dramatically in the next few decades. Because of the increase in the number of older adults, gerontologists increasingly call the extremes of this population the "young-old" (65–75 years) and the "old-aged" (85 years and older). Although every society seems to have a socially recognized category of "old person," definitions of what old age is can vary depending on time, place, and culture.

Old age increasingly is determined by the reaching of a specific chronological age, usually 65, because this represents the common time of retirement from the work force and the age at which pensions, such as Social Security, usually commence. Aging usually is defined chronologically but may depend on an array of *markers,* such as physical change, loss of certain abilities, or change in social roles.

DISEASES THAT AFFECT FOOT HEALTH IN OLDER ADULTS

Some diseases that rarely occur in younger people become increasingly common among people who are older than 65 years. Among them are cardiovascular diseases, such as arteriosclerosis, angina, other heart disease, and strokes, which are common causes of disability and death. Older adults also have a higher prevalence of cancer, especially prostate cancer, multiple myeloma, chronic lymphatic leukemia, lymphoma, and basal cell carcinoma. Chronic diseases that develop earlier in life also often present severe health problems in older adults because the metabolism becomes slower with age. For example, gangrene of the foot may occur in older adults with diabetes because of reduced circulation in the extremities. Some diseases are of special concern in older adults, such as bone disorders. Osteoporosis, or decrease in bone mass, mainly affects women after menopause; the bones become brittle, and even minor injuries can produce major fractures.

Also limited to older adults is Paget's disease, the slowly progressive deformation of bone. Osteoarthritis, which affects all older adults to some degree, can cause joint deformities, swelling, and pain. When the weight-bearing joints are affected, instability can result; this may be a cause of falling and fractures. Some degenerative neurological diseases, such as Parkinson's disease, occur almost exclusively among older adults, as does accidental hypothermia, the sudden drop in body temperature in response to cooler air temperatures, which is caused by age-related changes in the nervous system.

Mental disorders of physical or other origin also are a problem of old age. Dementia is a progressive deterioration of personality and intellect that can occur in the seventh and eighth decades of life. Several causes exist, including small vessel hemorrhages in the brain, viral infections of the brain, severe head injuries, tumors, alcoholism, vitamin deficiencies, pellagra, multiple sclerosis, and even lead or carbon monoxide poisoning. Alzheimer's disease, which is caused by deterioration of brain cells, has similar symptoms but usually begins in the fifth or sixth decade of life. In addition, depression in older adults can manifest symptoms that are almost identical to dementia; loss of interest in life, memory lapses, and living in the past are common in both conditions. Problems such as the loss of a spouse and the stress of living on a fixed income account for the high frequency of depression in older adults; the suicide rate among people who are older than 65 years is the second highest of any age group.

PODOGERIATRICS

Podogeriatrics is the special area of podiatric medicine that focuses on health promotion; prevention; and the treatment and management of foot and related problems, disability, deformity, and the pedal complications of chronic diseases in later life. Podogeriatrics is a component of health care for older adults. The Doctor of Podiatric Medicine who provides care for the older adult is trained to prevent and manage the unique and often multiple foot and related problems of older adults. These conditions may be local or the result of complications that are associated with multiple chronic diseases as well as the changes that are associated with the aging process itself.

Given that older adults tend to react to illness, deformity, and disease differently than do younger individuals, care includes an understanding of the specific syndromes that older adults experience and the complexity of being a part of a team that manages multiple diseases. In most cases, podogeriatric care is provided as part of a team approach to patient treatment, which involves many professionals. Under consideration for management is the individual's podiatric and medical history, present problems, the effects of both past illness and conditions and the current problems, and the individual's ability to participate in the development of care plans. Issues that relate to foot complaints also include their relationship to falls, confusion, neglect, and the capacity to perform the simple activities of daily living. Social support also is a consideration in patient care plans.

In many cases, because foot and related problems are the primary complaint, the individual seeks podiatric care initially. This entry into the health care system becomes the starting point for total geriatric care, with appropriate referrals. Comprehensive podogeriatric assessment is a component of this process.

Looking toward the future, there are many projections for the role of the podiatric practitioner. They include the knowledge and the ability to render care that not only is therapeutic in a medical sense but also provides comfort in a social sense. Podiatric practitioners also must recognize the importance of research in the field of aging, particularly as it relates to foot health. Significant areas include care delivery, biomechanics, behavior, and social aspects of immobility and methods to improve access to podiatry services in an attempt to improve the health of older adults.

The purpose of this training guide is to help long-term care (LTC) personnel better understand the need for foot health and podiatric care that is rendered to older adults and those who have ongoing health conditions and reside in LTC facilities. It can be used as a teaching guide for in-service education and as a self-teaching guide for all levels of personnel. This guide provides information on components of care: 1) assessment and 2) skin, nail, musculoskeletal, neurological, vascular, and systemic conditions that involve the foot, toes, and related areas. Some of the objectives of this training guide are to help professionals understand more about the care that is provided by the health care system, what should be considered in relation to the quality of care, and the alternative methods of care programs that are available in LTC. A glossary is included at the end of the book for the reader's reference.

CHAPTER ONE
Foot Health and Long-Term Care Facilities

F oot health long has been recognized as necessary for independent activity, individual dignity, and the general well-being of residents of long-term care (LTC) facilities. Problems that contribute to disability and pain lead to inactivity, listlessness, and deterioration of mental as well as physical health. By making LTC personnel aware of the many foot issues that arise in LTC residents, podogeriatric assessment and care can be instituted to prevent local foot problems and to minimize the complications that are associated with many ongoing health conditions and the effects of aging. In sharing this knowledge with LTC professionals, it is hoped that residents will benefit by receiving appropriate preventive measures as well as early intervention and care, thereby improving their quality of life.

Have you ever stopped to think how important your feet are in your daily activities? Imagine just for a moment how limited you would be if your feet were in such condition that you could not stand or walk without ongoing, unbearable pain or that you could not stand or walk at all. It has been demonstrated that by the time individuals reach 65 years of age, 95% will have developed some ongoing foot disorder that will require continuing assessment and management to permit them to stay active and productive. Feet are important and clearly require more attention as individuals grow older. This chapter addresses three basic issues: 1) the need for foot health, 2) the anatomy and properties of the foot, and 3) the role of podiatry in LTC facilities.

NEED FOR FOOT HEALTH

Before the LTC resident's need for foot care can be evaluated, LTC must be viewed in its entirety. The term *long-term care* once related only to geriatric institutions or facilities for those with mental disabilities, but the term has come to mean much more. Today, the term *long-term care* might broadly be defined as the management of any disease process, whether it be physical, functional, or mental, that requires extended care. That care may be institutionally based or modified to include some form of home care or life care. Individuals who are involved in LTC management, in or out of institutions, must have special knowledge about many unusual and complicated problems and the ability to adapt treatment methods to various circumstances.

The foot generally has received less attention than other parts of the human anatomy. There are common beliefs that as individuals age, feet are supposed to hurt and the ability to ambulate should decrease. The foot seldom is the cause of mortality but many times is the cause of morbidity, disease change, disability, and limited activity. Many signs of systemic disease may manifest first with foot symptoms. For example, an untreated diabetic ulcer that develops infection as a complication of diabetes may result in amputation or death.

If the resident of a LTC facility or institution is to function to the best of his or her ability, then he or she must be able to ambulate. This permits individuals to act for themselves, obtain their own food, maintain exercise programs, adjust their own television set, take care of their own personal needs, and, most important, maintain their dignity. Appropriate and indicated podiatric care and good foot health have four primary objectives in the LTC program: 1) to relieve pain, 2) to limit disability, 3) to restore a maximum level of independent activity, and 4) to prevent future complications from developing.

Many complications can result from inadequate assessment and foot care:

1. Loss of mobility

2. Increased discomfort and pain

3. Increase in complications that accompany ongoing health conditions

4. Likelihood of prolonged institutional care or bed confinement

5. Increase in the likelihood of hospitalization as a result of foot infection or a complication of peripheral arterial disease

Multiple studies (e.g., Gable, Haines, & Papp, 2004; Helfand, 2000, 2004; Helfand, Cooke, Walinksy, & Demp, 1998) have demonstrated that foot problems in LTC residents are widespread. In an assessment program in Pennsylvania, each patient had multiple foot complaints, and 75% reported pain at the time of evaluation. The assessment program also demonstrated that when foot problems were not managed appropriately and properly, early, simple foot problems became serious and required more intensive care, including hospitalization. Such problems can require so much care by nursing personnel that they might detract from care that is provided to other residents and significantly increase the cost of care. One study (Helfand, 1969) that was completed at an institution that is dedicated to the care of older adults with mental disabilities and did not have podiatric services before the assessment activity revealed that the residents' foot health improved or stabilized, costs were reduced, and the quality of life of the residents improved when podiatric services were added. Even though the patients grew older, ongoing health conditions progressed, and the potential for complications increased, appropriate foot care helped to prevent the development of new foot problems. This was the largest such study completed at that time and still stands as the largest study almost 40 years later.

The foot is an efficient structure of propulsion and locomotion as well as the static foundation of the upright stance. Through the years, it must carry a physical workload that is exceeded only by organs such as the heart and the lungs. The human foot is a flexible organ that was not designed to walk on modern civilization's hard, flat surfaces. As individuals age and proceed through their working years, the physical abuse of weight and repetitive stress and injury change the anatomic structure and functioning of the foot. Adding "risk diseases"—that is, ongoing health conditions and their complications, such as arthritis, diabetes, and peripheral arterial and neurological diseases—places the older adult at risk for developing serious foot problems that can limit mobility and alter in a negative manner the quality of life.

ANATOMY AND PROPERTIES OF THE FOOT

The human foot is complex (see Figure 1). Each foot has 26 bones (together constituting one fourth of the body's total) plus ossicles, ligaments, muscles, tendons, arteries, veins, nerves, and, of course, its covering of skin. The muscles are attached to specific parts of the foot by tendons, which are elastic and cause movement when the muscles contract. More than 100 ligaments hold the structures together. The long plantar ligament, situated on the bottom of each foot, is the strongest and acts as a trampoline to absorb shock and support body weight. The foot normally bears weight on a triangular base with the long sides being the inner and outer borders of the foot, or longitudinal arches, and the short side being the bias along the five metatarsal bone heads, just proximal to or behind the toes. The arches, which are the main springs, or shock absorbers, are key parts of the foot's design. Each spring consists of a row of bones, strong ligaments, muscle, cartilage, and joints.

Feet are designed to perform two major functions: support and mobility. The heel of the foot serves as a firm pedestal for standing. Weight is transferred from the calcaneus, or heel bone, to the first and fifth metatarsals at the base of the toes. The toes and the front of the foot are used primarily to push in the off phase of walking (phases include heel strike, support, heel off, toe off, and swing). The flexibility and the strength of feet affect how a person walks, which in turn affects posture and how a person carries his or her weight. Neglected feet, which become stiff or weak, can cause backache, leg cramps, fatigue, and loss of balance; place a person at greater risk for a fall; re-

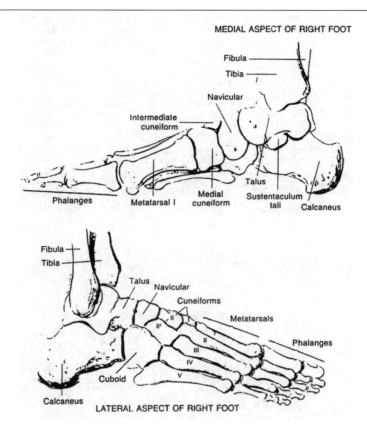

Figure 1. Anatomy of the foot. (From Pedorthic Footwear Association. [n.d.]. *Pedorthic reference guide*. Columbia, MD: Author. Copyright © Pedorthic Footwear Association, Columbia, MD, 1992, 1999, 2006. All rights reserved. Reprinted with permission.)

duce a person's ability to ambulate; and diminish a person's quality of life.

A normal foot in an older person cannot be defined anatomically. By the time a person is defined as being a senior citizen, some deformity has taken place. The skin has undergone changes; the bones have deviated, or shifted; the muscles have demonstrated some wasting; and some limitation of motion has occurred. Significant changes occur in toenails of older adults; they become thickened and brittle and do not resemble the toenails of people in younger age groups. They are misshapen or diseased and may produce pain and limitation of function, but they can be managed properly, usually with conservative care.

The basic structure of the foot is bone. The talus, with the lower portions of the leg bones (tibia and fibula), makes up part of the ankle joint. The talus has no muscular attachments; therefore, the tendons and muscles that parallel the talus control activity.

Beneath the talus is the heel bone. It is a much larger bone and is attached to the Achilles tendon in the posterior, or rear, segment. It is a major contributor to foot function. Anterior to, or in front of, the heel bone is the cuboid, a rectangular-shaped bone that adds to the structural support of the foot. In front of the talus is the navicular, a coin-shaped bone that also provides muscular attachments. In front of the navicular and lateral, or adjacent, to the cuboid are three wedge-shaped bones called the first, second, and third cuneiforms. They help to provide stability to the foot. These bones make up the *rear foot.*

In front of the cuneiforms and cuboid bones are the five metatarsals. Each metatarsal consists of a base, a shaft, and a head. They are anatomically classed as long bones. In front of the metatarsals are the phalanges. Each of the smaller toes contains three phalanges; the great toe is composed of two phalanges.

Each bone that attaches to another forms a joint. Bones are attached to each other by a series of ligaments, or fibrous bands, that hold them together. Their functional role is to maintain proximity, or to keep the segments of bone close to each other. Their properties are strength and rigidity with limited elasticity, which permits the joints to maintain some degree of motion or movement.

The ligamentous attachments of all of the bones are numerous. They generally include ligaments on the top (superior), on the bottom (inferior), and to the sides (medial and lateral), depending on the joint. Ligaments do not attach to the segments of bone that touch each other to form the articular surfaces. These surfaces are covered with cartilage. There are stronger joints and weaker joints, but one crucial point in understanding foot anatomy is that each toe joint has what are called membranous expansions so that the attachments of muscles and ligaments truly bind together in a firm manner all of the joints to each toe. These expansions permit all of the muscles in the foot to aid in its propulsive activity.

Bone changes that occur in aging might be defined as a loss of mineral substance (i.e., primarily calcium) and may clinically be termed *osteopenia* or *osteoporosis*. Radiographs, or X-ray films, demonstrate a washed out appearance of the bones and may be termed *eggshell* in appearance. This usually means that the cortex, or outer segment of the bone, still remains white but that the medulla, or inner component of the bone, appears clear or washed out. This results in a weakening of bone itself. A common fracture that occurs as a result of this weakening, coupled with a twisting or bending of tissue without evidence or a history of trauma (injury), is called a pathologic, or stress, fracture.

The basic change in foot ligaments as a result of aging is the transition from elasticity to rigidity. A ligament that binds one bone to another is strong; it takes force to sever it. When a ligament is pulled away from bone, it generally pulls some of the bone cells with it, causing a sprain, which, if severe, can be worse than a fracture. There is less chance of healing once this occurs.

The most predominant and significant membranous covering of the foot is called the *plantar fascia*. It attaches to the posterior, or back, segment of the heel bone at a segment of the heel that is known as the tuberosity and fans out forward into the metatarsal area, just under the skin, on the plantar, or bottom, surface of the foot. The plantar fascia covers all of the foot muscles, all of the ligaments, and all of the bones on the bottom of the foot. It acts as a spring to aid in function and protects all of the structures on the bottom of the foot. It is a very elastic or flexible mass in youth, which becomes less flexible and rigid with age.

The dorsum, or the top part, of the foot does not have such a strong fascial attachment. In fact, most of the structures are just beneath the skin. Therefore, any severe trauma or injury to the top of the foot tends to be more of a problem than an injury on the bottom of the foot.

Many of the muscles that guide the foot originate in the leg. On the top surface of the foot, they include the tendon that controls the great toe (extensor hallucis longus) and four tendons that control the lesser toes (extensor digitorum longus). These tendons function to dorsiflex the foot, or turn the foot upward. In addition, a shorter tendon and ligament (tibialis anterior) arises from the medial, or inner, portion of the leg and functions to turn the foot medially, or inward. The tendons on the lateral, or outside, portion of the foot (peroneus longus and peroneus brevis) arise from the lateral portion of the leg and permit the foot to be pulled laterally, or outward. The muscles that arise from the top of the foot (extensor digitorum hallucis brevis and digitorum brevis) help to pull the foot toward the leg. A decrease in muscle strength can be seen in older adults and those with ongoing health conditions. This can result in a foot drop, a condition whereby stronger extending muscles on the bottom of the foot overpower those on the top of the foot.

The nerves that control the foot come from the spinal cord by way of the sciatic nerve in the leg. Through branches, it supplies both the upper and the lower portions of the foot. The nerves on the bottom of the foot include the lateral plantar nerve and the medial plantar nerve. They subdivide into branches and supply all of the toes with both sensation and function. On the top portion of the foot, the superficial nerves provide the same function. The saphenous nerve supplies the inner segment of the foot, and the sural nerve supplies the outer segment of the toe area.

The blood vessels of the foot also come from the leg, each branching off from a larger blood vessel. The main arteries of the foot are close to the bones. They include the major artery on the top of the foot (dorsalis pedis), which usually can be palpated just beside the tendon that leads to the great toe. This major artery then subdivides into metatarsal and digital arteries and then into capillaries.

The major artery on the bottom surface of the foot (posterior tibial) also is close to bone, thereby affording protection to the vital blood supply. This artery can be palpated just behind the inner portion of the ankle. It provides more blood to the foot than does the artery on the top of the foot. This also subdivides into metatarsal arteries and supplies blood to the toes.

The function of the blood vessels is to transport blood to the foot. The changes that blood vessels undergo during the aging process are especially important. Because of the accumulation of fatty material (plaque) inside the arteries (arteriosclerosis), blood flow to the foot decreases. When blood flow is blocked, the development of gangrene, or death, of a part of the foot can follow. Complicating diseases, such as diabetes, contribute to development of arteriosclerotic complications, which places the individual at greater risk for amputation.

The skin of the foot is made up of fitted, flexible, elastic inner dermis that is covered by a much less sensitive outer epidermis. The skin varies in thickness from 0.5 millimeter (mm) in the eyelid to 4 or 5 mm in the sole of the foot. The skin of the foot undergoes many changes during the aging process. It becomes thinner, even parchment like; loses its elasticity; usually atrophies; and loses hair. It loses its hydration because there generally is less perspiration and lubrication. The skin loses its suppleness, becomes brittle and dry, and injures easily. This condition, accompanied by a diminished blood supply, can be serious.

ROLE OF PODIATRY IN LONG-TERM CARE FACILITIES

Because the foot is such a specialized structure, licensed practitioners in a special discipline, podiatric medicine, are the primary providers of care of the human foot and its related structures. With their colleagues in the other health disciplines, such as medicine, osteopathic medicine, and dentistry, podiatrists are educated, trained, and licensed by law to prescribe and treat conditions of the foot medically and surgically. In LTC facilities, the podiatrist usually functions in the role of a consultant; the admitting and attending physician (M.D. or D.O.) has the primary role of managing the individual's overall medical condition. The podiatric service functions in concert with the medical service not only to treat deformities and diseases of the foot but also to manage the complications of related systemic diseases and, perhaps equally important, to provide the concept of prevention, which are the keys to good foot health and to maintaining a good quality of life.

In addition to patient consultation and care, the podiatrist may function as a health educator by providing formal or informal and practical in-service educational programs for nurses, nursing assistants, and related staff. Consulting podiatrists also should be involved in administrative decisions related to foot health and care and patient management conferences. Patient education also can be supplemented for both patients and family. Foot health is accomplished by a team effort. Everyone can play an important role, as foot health and foot care are extremely important to the individual's total health, especially for the older adult and individuals with ongoing health conditions. Foot health is important to maintaining the LTC resident's mobility and dignity.

CHAPTER TWO

Improving Early Recognition of Foot Problems in the Long-Term Care Resident

Clinical Podogeriatric Assessment

The early detection and treatment of health problems are of paramount importance in preventive health practices, but many times this concept is diminished when it concerns the feet. Feet are not supposed to hurt, so when they do, attention should be paid to them. Because many complications of systemic diseases have their first onset in the foot, appropriate assessment is a critical element in comprehensive health care of older adults.

Much of the ability to remain ambulatory throughout the stages of aging is related directly to foot health. To maintain foot health, practitioners must think comprehensively and recognize that team care must be an essential part of the management of ongoing health conditions in the care of the older adult. It is clear that adults with ongoing health conditions and older adults are at high risk for foot-related disease and should continue foot assessment, education, surveillance, and care. For this group of individuals, the ability to prevent complications and maintain mobility and ambulation will be reflected in their quality of life and their ability to remain mentally alert and active in their communities.

This chapter is designed to educate nurses, nursing assistants, and others in long-term care (LTC) facilities about the specifics of early detection of common foot disorders among older adults and those with ongoing health conditions. These key personnel must use their expertise, knowledge, powers of observation, and daily contact with residents to detect problems and report them to the attending physician and consulting podiatrist. Reviewed are the primary components of residents' histories, physical examination of the foot, interpretation of various foot complaints, and help in identifying the difference between normal and abnormal findings as basic tools in the everyday contact with LTC residents.

COMPREHENSIVE PODOGERIATRIC ASSESSMENT

The role of LTC staff in detecting and preventing foot disorders is important. One important tool that is available and a part of the resident's record is the medical history and the family history. The history should contain information on the resident's present and past disease, physical condition, and a comprehensive review of the medical problems that are prevalent in the individual's family. The history also should include the resident's former address, which may relate to environmental influence that may affect the medical condition. Hereditary and racial background should be noted for similar reasons. The patient's age is important; changes occur in the aging foot, and what may be normal in younger individuals may differ in older adults, particularly in relation to foot function. However, age is not a determining factor alone. The ages of family members also are important, as are ages and causes of death of deceased family members. Finally, the history should contain a record of social habits, such as smoking, drinking, and substance abuse. Present and past medications, including over-the-counter preparations, are important factors to be identified. Smoking directly affects the circulatory system by constricting blood vessels, thereby reducing blood flow. Excessive alcohol consumption can lead to numbness of the feet or neuropathy in addition to problems in other body systems.

Foot health and foot care are important and often overlooked components of an older person's overall health and well-being, because some foot pain is considered normal. Foot problems may hinder a person's ability to be free of pain and discomfort, to maintain proper mobility, to enjoy interpersonal relationships, to have a positive self-image, and to maintain activity and independence and a high quality of life. Many ongoing health conditions, such as diabetes, peripheral arterial insufficiency, arthritis, other metabolic diseases and conditions that produce pain, vascular limitations, and diminished sensation, are more prevalent in older adults, and symptoms increase as individuals age. These individuals are at higher risk for ongoing complications and comorbidities, which increase the potential for marked limitation of activity, hospitalization, and limb loss.

Foot health is related directly to older adults' being able to maintain their activities of daily living and it contributes to the development of conditions that are associated with disability, such as arthritis and ulceration. Foot problems are common in older adults as a result of disease, deformity, complications, and neglect that results from a lack of preventive service at the primary, secondary, and tertiary levels. They contribute to disability and can reduce an older person's independence and quality of life.

Medicare may provide coverage for what is defined as primary "foot and nail care" or "routine foot care" if the criteria of vascular and sensory deficits are met. There are systemic conditions that permit coverage; see the Appendix at the end of the book for detailed information.

Many other factors also contribute to the development of foot problems of older adults, including the aging process itself and abuse and neglect. Some of these considerations include the following:

- Degree of ambulation
- Duration of previous hospitalization
- Limitation of activity
- Previous institutionalization

- Episodes of social segregation
- Previous care
- Emotional adjustments to disease and life in general
- Multiple medications and drug interactions
- Complications and residuals associated with risk diseases

We have established that knowledge of the individual's background, medical history, family history, age, gender, and social habits can be a great aid to the LTC staff in detecting a potential problem for the individual. Heredity, environment, nutrition, and social habits all contribute to the development of foot problems in the older adult.

Observing and Examining in an Ongoing Fashion

Perhaps more important to the nursing staff than the family and personal history are the constant observation, assessment, and examination of the feet of the individual. Each time the individual is assisted with bathing, dressing, feeding, walking, or exercising, the staff member should be observing him or her for skin changes, skin abrasions and/or ulcers, painful joints, and other problems, particularly in the feet and the legs.

One of the first things to notice is the color of the skin. In the older adult, the skin color may be pale to red to reddish-blue. Skin that is marble white usually is associated with pain and numbness. This may indicate an acute vascular insufficiency, which many times is a medical emergency. Color changes that affect only one foot also are very important. Areas of dark pigmentation over major arteries may indicate circulatory deficits or early clotting. Red spots in areas of pressure on the bottom of the foot can be a precursor to ulceration, especially in individuals with diabetes. Black or blue moles that change in color, enlarge, or bleed may indicate early malignancy. Variations in the texture of the skin (smooth, rough, glossy, dull, pigmented, scaly, clear, or parchment like) are helpful, if recognized, in determining the presence of circulatory disease, dermatological problems, and other systemic conditions.

Swelling, pain, hyperkeratotic lesions (heloma [corn] and tyloma [callus]), and toenail changes also need to be observed. Some of the

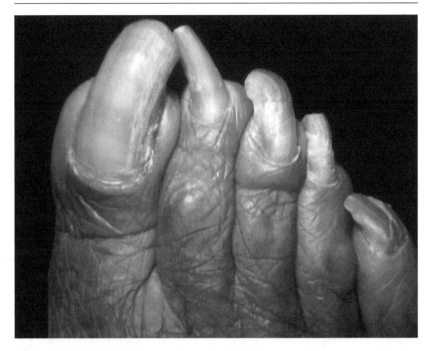

Figure 2. Abnormal nail curvature (onychodysplasia) with thickened nail plate (onychauxis) and fungal infection (onychomycosis).

more common toenail changes in the older adult include thickening (onychauxis), severe deformity and growth (onychogryphosis), abnormal curvature (onychodysplasia), ingrown toenails (onychocryptosis), inflammation (onychia), infection (paronychia), and fungal infection (onychomycosis). Xerosis (dryness) and the presence of ulceration also should be noted (see Figures 2–4 for examples).

Checking the temperature of the foot is a good diagnostic procedure. The normal foot temperature varies between 92° Fahrenheit (F) and 98° F and may be determined by a skin thermometer or radiometer. Touching both feet at the same time provides an indication of relative foot temperature. Disparity is what is important to notice. Excessive warmth of one foot may indicate an inflammation or an infection. Coldness in one foot may mean clinical evidence of inadequate or poor arterial circulation or a neurological deficit affecting the vascular system. Excessive perspiration may indicate a nervous system problem, faulty foot mechanics, pain, or dermatological problems,

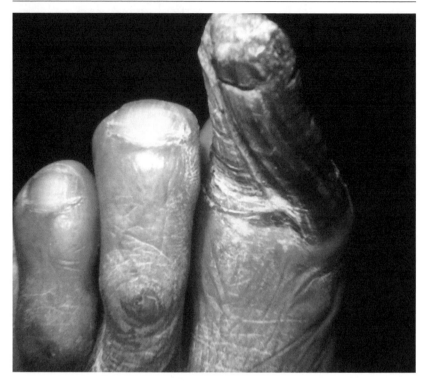

Figure 3. Severe toenail deformity (onychogryphosis) with fungal infection (onychomycosis).

such as a fungal infection. Emotional disturbances and allergic reactions also can precipitate excessive perspiration. Temperature changes in each individual toe can be determined, especially in individuals with diabetes. If one toe is colder than the others, then this could signify a local vascular deficit that could lead to gangrene and possible amputation if not identified and treated promptly.

Checking pulses in the foot and the leg is important. Each foot has two pulses, one on the top of the foot (dorsalis pedis) and the other behind the medial, or innermost part of the ankle (posterior tibial). The dorsalis pedis usually is palpable, or can be felt, just lateral to the tendon that extends to the great toe. Occasionally, the pulse on the dorsum, or top, of the foot may not be palpable and a Doppler study may be needed to locate the anatomic position of the pulse. The posterior tibial pulse, just behind the inner portion of the ankle, usually is palpable, except in cases of decreased circulation. It

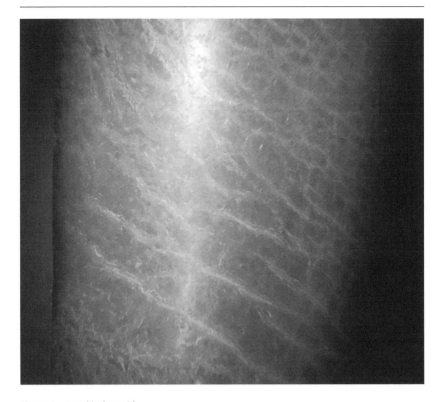

Figure 4. Dry skin (xerosis).

is best to palpate the pulses with the middle three fingers to minimize the chances of recording one's own pulse. There also is a pulse behind the knee, the popliteal pulse, which can be felt by holding the knee from the front with thumbs placed on the kneecap and fingers exerting mild pressure behind the knee. With practice, one will be able to find these pulses and differentiate normal from abnormal. There also is a femoral pulse in the groin, should all other lower extremity pulses not be palpable.

The rate of the pulse is not as important as the strength and the fullness of the pulses for both feet. Questions to ask include the following: Are they equally as strong? If not, then should there be additional investigation and consultation? Other symptoms and signs of circulatory change (peripheral arterial disease) include coldness, trophic changes, night cramps, edema or swelling, claudication (pain in the calf during walking), and varicosities associated with venous disease.

Other means of examination, such as checking blood pressures in both the leg and the arm, can be valuable in diagnosing problems such as vascular insufficiency, aortic insufficiency, and coarctation of the aorta. Like the pulse, blood pressure readings should be observed for equal strength. If a wide disparity occurs, then further investigation should be initiated.

Determining the presence or absence of tendon reflexes also may be helpful. The knee reflex is elicited by striking the patellar tendon, just below the kneecap, with the knee bent. The same procedure is performed posterior to, or behind, the ankle joint with the Achilles tendon. The lack of reflexes or the increased force of a reflex may be the earliest sign of neurological disease. Other aspects to examine include the vibratory sense, areas where there is a loss of sensation or protective sensation, response to sharp and dull pressure or heat and cold, joint position, the superficial plantar reflex (Babinski), and burning or abnormal sensations (neuropathy).

Foot deformities should be noted. Some of the most common in the older adult include hallux valgus (bunion deformity), anterior imbalance, metatarsal prolapse, soft tissue atrophy, digiti flexus (hammertoe), pes planus or pes valgo planus (lowering of the medial longitudinal or inner arch), pes cavus (extremely high arched foot), hallux rigidus or limitus (arthritis of the great toe joint), Morton's syndrome (short first metatarsal segment), tailor's bunion (bunionette of the fifth metatarsal phalangeal joint), and excessive deformity with sensory change in individuals with diabetes (Charcot joints or foot) (see Figures 5–7 for examples).

Manual muscle testing is another important procedure that is used in diagnosing foot problems or conditions. Simply applying pressure to each of the four sides of the foot and having the individual then exert an opposite force can accomplish this. This provides a relative indication of the strength of the person's individual leg muscles and provides an early indicator of balance changes and possible fall risk problems.

Investigating Complaints of Foot Pain and Other Sensations

Although some of the primary physical indicators of foot problems have been identified, one very important intangible indicator is pain. When the individual complains of pain, burning, or itching, it always

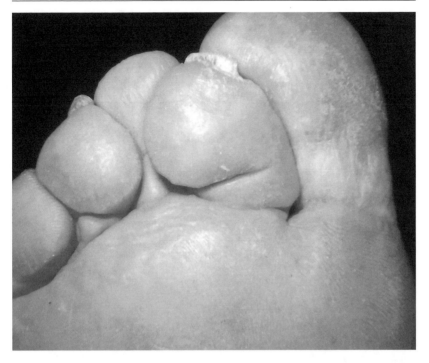

Figure 5. Bunion deformity (hallux valgus) with toe joint deformity (prolapsed second toe with rotation).

should be examined and investigated. That the individual may be older and at times incoherent or exhibiting cognitive impairment should not prevent the staff from listening to and acting on any complaint.

Foot pain is a common complaint, especially in older adults. As a person ages, joints become arthritic, arterial circulation decreases, muscles become wasted, and the chances of injury and damage to the foot and the leg increase. Even simple problems can become complicated. For example, a heloma (corn) or a tyloma (callus) on the bottom of the foot may cause the patient to limp and favor that foot, thereby shifting weight abnormally and causing other problems to develop. This change in balance places the patient at risk for falling. Pain may be reported as cramping; burning; dull aching; tingling; or sharp, shooting pains.

Cramping is a common complaint that usually is caused by an unnatural position of or impaired arterial circulation in the foot. Cramps in the foot and the leg while in bed, during sleep, or while walking

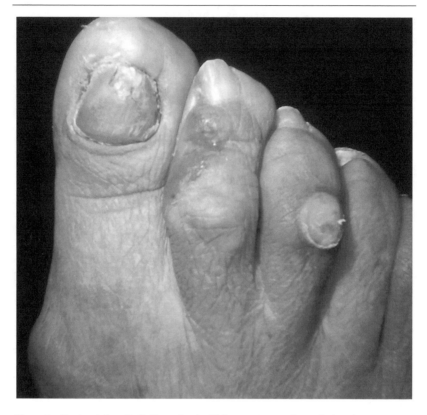

Figure 6. Bunion deformity (hallux valgus) with hammertoes and corn (heloma).

(intermittent claudication) can signify arterial insufficiency. Deformities and nutritional deficiencies also can cause cramping.

A complaint of tingling or numbness and burning can be caused by many disorders. A nerve tumor (neuroma) between two toes can cause tingling in those toes and burning between the toes. Compression of the sciatic nerve in the back can cause tingling in the heel and the back of the leg. Numbness and a loss of sensation can be caused by nerve irritation, vascular insufficiency, or such systemic diseases as diabetes or ongoing alcoholism. Vitamin deficiencies, anemia, and dietary problems also are common causes of tingling and burning.

Soreness can be due to overworked muscles, stretched ligaments and joints, and inflammation of veins (phlebitis) in the leg. A common complaint in the older adult is soreness on the top or the inside of the great toe. This may be related to arthritis, arteriosclerosis, neuritis, or shoe compression.

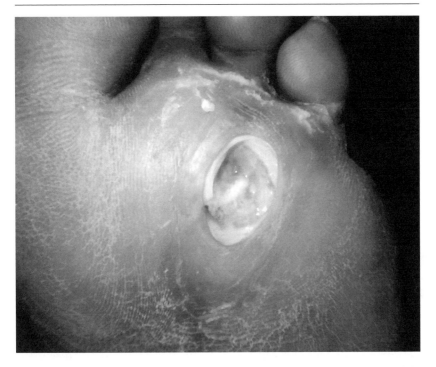

Figure 7. Avascular diabetic ulcer.

Sharp, shooting pains may be caused by a nerve that is entrapped or a fracture of a bone in the foot. If it occurs on arising and stepping out of bed in the morning, then it may be due to arthritis. The possibility of a pathologic fracture of a bone in the foot always should be considered, with appropriate imaging studies completed as indicated.

Just as important as the complaint of pain, however, is the situation in which an obvious condition exists but elicits no complaint. Ulcers on the foot that are not painful should arouse suspicion in the LTC professional. These may be caused by diabetes or other systemic diseases and should be evaluated and managed properly. Many older adults, because of embarrassment or modesty or not wanting to be a bother or a burden, will not complain of problems, or they believe that their feet are ugly and do not like to show them. Many people believe that feet are supposed to hurt all the time, especially in older adults. In addition, it is common that a problem will be present but the person will not feel pain or will be unaware of sensation changes. Circulatory deficiencies and diseases such as diabetes can cause a gradual loss of sensation that precludes or masks pain. This is an especially dangerous situation and further adds to the importance of the staff members' implementing all examination techniques. See the Appendix at the end of the book for an explanation of a comprehensive assessment protocol.

CONCLUSION

Foot impairment, including diseases and disorders of the foot, are common in older adults and may affect a person's general health and functioning. Periodic comprehensive podogeriatric assessment is recommended for older adults. Staff members need to be aware of local conditions and the complications of systemic diseases, such as diabetes, peripheral arterial disease, arthritic changes, neurological deficiencies, and mental health symptoms, that manifest foot symptoms and signs. Staff members should recognize the common clinical findings and should refer individuals for podiatric care and management in a timely and appropriate manner as indicated. Inasmuch as a majority of geriatric foot problems cannot be totally prevented, the concept of secondary prevention, i.e., finding the disorder or disease at its earliest manifestation and managing the disorder properly, can significantly improve the quality of life for older adults.

CHAPTER THREE

Identifying and Caring for Common Skin and Nail Problems in the Long-Term Care Resident

Duuring the course of a lifetime, the human foot endures much use, misuse, abuse, trauma, and neglect. The stress of daily activity, the constant enclosure of the foot, and the degenerative changes of aging all are issues that must be considered in keeping an individual ambulatory. Foot discomfort and pain in older adults can significantly reduce the quality of life and mobility, thereby reducing independence.

Given this information, it is easy to understand that a vast number of common local, chronic foot problems are those of the skin and toenails. This chapter reviews some of the common foot complaints that are associated with these areas. This initial segment focuses on some of the common skin problems that are associated with long-term care (LTC) residents.

SKIN PROBLEMS

The skin of the older adult's foot is noticeably different from that of a younger person. It is less supple than youthful skin because of diminished elasticity of the fibers beneath the epidermis and the dermis. There may be a loss of hair on the outer side of the leg and the foot, distinctive brownish pigmentation changes, dryness, scaling, and atrophy. This dryness is associated with naturally diminishing oily secretions, dehydration, and atrophy. Other changes are due to metabolic and nutritional factors.

Common dermatological (skin and toenail) problems in the feet of older adults and those with ongoing health conditions are varied, and because of the delicate nature of the individual's condition, treatment usually is approached initially in a conservative manner. The exceptions include significant infection, life-threatening events, and the potential for malignancy. An individual often is admitted to an LTC facility with ongoing foot conditions. The problems in treating these individuals are multiple. Future problems as well as complications in the existing condition must be prevented.

Structure and Composition of the Foot's Skin

The skin consists of the epidermis (outer layer) which varies in thickness, and the dermis (inner layer). The outermost layer of the epidermis (stratum corneum) consists of cells that contain keratin, a fibrous protein. It is thickest where external trauma is greatest, such as the soles of the feet. This stratum corneum actually increases in thickness with trauma or repetitive injury. The outer layers peel off as new cells are formed continuously to maintain this thickness. The deeper layer of the stratum corneum serves as a barrier to absorption of substances through the skin. The dermis (corium) is the inner section of the skin and contains blood vessels; nerves; and such tissues as sweat glands, ducts, and hair follicles and their sebaceous glands.

The nerve supply of the skin conducts both sensory and motor impulses. The sensory nerves transmit the perception of touch, temperature, and pain. The motor nerves control sweat glands, arterioles, and the smooth muscle of the skin. The most common presenting symptoms include painful or painless wounds; slow-healing or non-healing wounds; trophic ulceration; necrosis; skin color changes such as cyanosis or redness, changes in texture, or turgor; pigmentation related to hemosiderin deposition; chronic itching; scaling; excessive dryness, or xerosis; diminished or absent hair growth; and atrophy or a parchment-like appearance.

Hyperkeratotic Lesions

Hyperkeratotic lesions usually result from repetitive minimal trauma over extended periods, continuing frictions, deformity, gait change, and pressure on the skin, which cause an abnormally thickened mass of keratin. The term *hyperkeratotic* means overactive production of keratotic tissue, without any real change in function. The most common hyperkeratotic lesions are forms of tyloma (callus) and heloma (corn). Calluses often occur over a bony enlargement or at a site of abnormal weight distribution. Corns usually are found about the toes and commonly are caused by pressure that is associated with inappropriate foot-to-footwear relationships or by bony prominences. Shoes are constructed over a model, or last. When the shape of the shoe, or the last, does not conform to the shape of the foot, excessive pressure is generated. It is like trying to place a square peg into a round hole.

The two most common forms of corn are the hard corn (heloma durum) and soft corn (heloma molle). The hard corn usually is found on the top surface of the toes, on the outer sides of the first and fifth metatarsal phalangeal joints, or on the bottom surface of the foot at sites of excessive pressure. The soft corn differs from the hard corn in that it absorbs perspiration and moisture because it usually is found between the toes. Another lesion is the heloma neurofibrosum, which contains a central portion of fibrous and nerve tissue. This form of heloma is especially painful, with a throbbing, burning, and stabbing pain, and is found in an area of extreme pressure or at the site of direct trauma. It can be recognized by an irregular outline and a white or gray color. These lesions sometimes are referred to as intractable keratosis and may be related to eccrine poroma (plugged sweat gland).

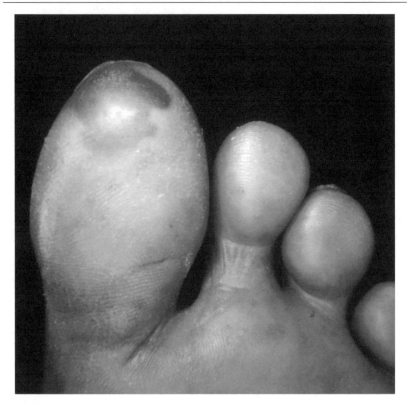

Figure 8. Diabetic hematoma.

Heloma vasculare is like heloma durum, but the abnormally thick-ened tissue also has elements of hemorrhage and may bleed easily when debrided. Its orange and red to yellow linear discolorations are separated by a callus and covered with a dry or moist tissue. The pres-ence of a hematoma, or hemorrhage, beneath a callus or a corn may be the first sign of an ulcer, especially in older adults who have dia-betes (Figure 8).

Miliary helomas usually consist of multiple localized spotty areas of hyperkeratosis that measure approximately 1 to 3millimeters in di-ameter. They are multiple and deeply imbedded and appear nearly white to yellow in color, resembling the head of a small brass nail.

Calluses look different depending on the part of the foot (includ-ing the heel and the toes) on which they occur. They can be extremely painful and seem to be more diffuse than corns.

Calluses and corns can be treated in a conservative manner but may require surgical revision if there are severe bony prominences or deformity involved. Treatment depends on the cause, size, location of the callus or corn and the individual's health and age. Both must be treated judiciously because they are capable of developing complications, such as infection and ulceration. The initial treatment and management includes local debridement to reduce the thickness of the keratosis, the use of emollients, and procedures to reduce and modify pressure to the involved area. This can be accomplished by a change in footwear and by the prescription of an orthotic or digital device. Orthotics usually are constructed of a variety of materials, including leather, rubber, synthetic closed- and open-cell foams, silicone, felt, and other materials to shield painful areas. Dispersing pressure from the painful area and diffusing pressure usually are considerations in management. Patient education also is a key element in management, as is as an avoidance of over-the-counter preparations that use acid to reduce hyperkeratosis.

Another common foot complaint, more prevalent in younger individuals, is warts, or verrucae. Warts are caused by a virus, and there are many types. When present on the bottom of the foot, they are referred to as plantar warts. Another type, mosaic verruca (Figure 9), consists of numerous warts that coalesce to form a larger lesion that resembles mosaic tiles. Verrucae are benign and cause pain, particularly on weight-bearing surfaces, and keratosis is noted. Irritation and ongoing health conditions add to the discomfort. Management includes surgical excision; electrical destruction; cryotherapy, or freezing; and chemical destruction. Removing pressure from the area helps to reduce the pain.

Disorders of the Sweat Glands

Disorders of the sweat glands include hyperhidrosis, an abnormal increase of perspiration, and anhidrosis, an abnormal decrease in perspiration. When a fetid odor (foul smell) is noted with excessive perspiration, it is known as bromidrosis and is associated with bacterial decomposition of the perspiration. In addition, excessive perspiration increases the potential for fungal infection, or tinea pedis. Maceration (moisture) also may be present. The causes of excessive perspi-

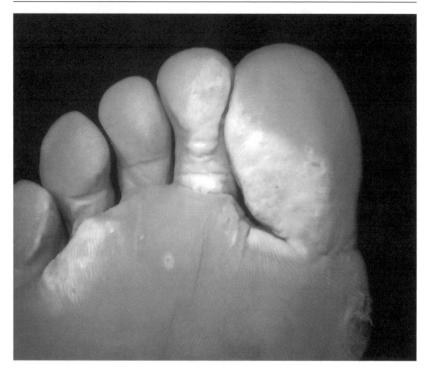

Figure 9. Wart mass (mosaic verruca).

ration may be metabolic, neurological, nutritional, or allergic or may be related to shoes and stockings. With anhidrosis, the skin begins to fissure, or crack. Treatment of these conditions depends on the cause and normalizing the functions of the sweat glands, as well as the general physical status of the individual.

With excessive perspiration, the patient should wear hosiery that can absorb moisture. Material with a weave that is wide enough to allow for evaporation is preferred. Lightweight woolen hose or quality cotton or synthetic fibers that have a wicking effect are recommended. Synthetic substances, such as nylon or Orlon, usually do not permit adequate evaporation of excessive perspiration and may cause the skin to become soggy, irritated, macerated, and painful. Hosiery with cotton soles and heels is an alternative. Poorly constructed and ill-fitting shoes also may be a contributing factor, and those that are constructed with plastic and rubber compounds tend to prevent

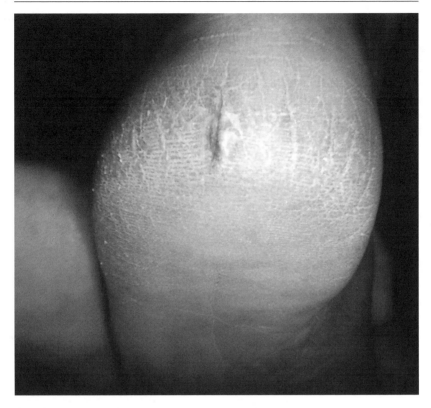

Figure 10. Heel fissure.

evaporation. Cleanliness, topical astringents, and appropriate dusting powders that absorb perspiration are indicated. In the early stages of odor, topical powders that contain neomycin can help to reduce bacterial decomposition of perspiration.

Anhidrosis is the abnormally low output of perspiration. It may be caused either by sluggish sweat glands or by mechanical obstruction of the sweat gland ducts and pores. This limits the normal excretion of perspiration and causes the skin to be dry, scaly, cracked, and sometimes parchment-like. Cleanliness is equally important, as is the local and systemic management of the problem. The use of emollients and moisturizing agents is suggested. One possible complication of anhidrosis is fissured heels (Figure 10). The skin cracks and develops a fissure or an ulceration. Fissured heels can be serious when there is an associated poor blood supply to the heel. The broken skin is more susceptible to infection. Therapy is directed to closing the fissures and at future prevention.

Fungal Infections

Fungal, or mycotic, infections are another skin condition that can occur in LTC residents. Tinea pedis, or athlete's foot, usually presents with itching, scaling, redness, and maceration, particularly between the toes. If not recognized and managed early, secondary bacterial infection can develop. In the older adult, this complication can be more serious than in younger individuals because of the presence of ongoing health conditions such as diabetes and peripheral arterial insufficiency. In addition, the older adult who has diminished or loss of sensation or has difficulty in bending or even seeing one's own feet may not complain about these conditions. Management includes a variety of topical medications, such as solutions, creams, and ointments, depending on the presentation, and the use of an appropriate foot powder as a preventive measure. Cleanliness, stocking, and footwear considerations also are key elements in total management and prevention. Fungal skin infections also predispose individuals to fungal infections of the toenails and vice versa. Other infections include pyoderma, cellulitis (Figure 11), and toenail infections, such as onychomycosis and paronychia. Bacterial infections, such as those noted, require appropriate antibiotics and result in early complications if not managed properly.

Contact Dermatitis

Contact dermatitis is another dermatological problem that presents in older adults. Any material or topical medication, in particular, can precipitate skin changes. Shoe dyes, shoe linings, insole material, or foot covering material, such as stockings or shoes, can precipitate an event. Symptoms usually include an area of limited and circumscribed inflammation, with a possible history of allergy. There are shoe test kits to help with identification of the allergic agent, which may be the nickel in the shoe dye. The primary irritant (allergic component) must be isolated and removed. Management and treatment are directed toward the skin symptoms and changes and may include mild astringent or saline compresses and topical steroids.

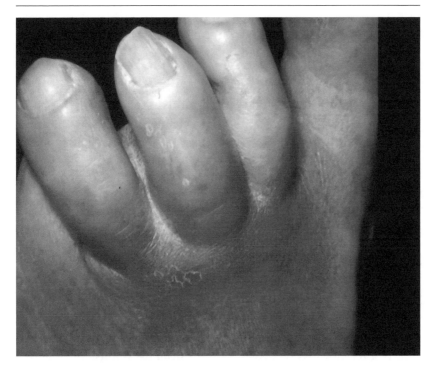

Figure 11. Shedding of skin (cellulitis).

Ulcers

Ulcers are the result of external problems, systemic disease, or a combination of these factors. Ulceration results from external causes such as trauma; decubitus ulceration (bed sores); trophic changes; scratches from excessive itching; and burns—thermal, electrical, or chemical (e.g., those caused by strong acids in over-the-counter preparations). The internal or systemic diseases that can cause ulceration include arterial or venous insufficiencies, diabetes, gout, and the residuals of sexually transmitted diseases. Treatment depends on the cause and may include imaging (e.g., X-rays, magnetic resonance imaging scans), antibiotics, chemical debriding agents, pressure reduction, physical medicine, surgical debridement, topical dressings, compresses, meticulous wound care, and ambulatory aids. The key is to make the appropriate diagnosis, to manage it early, to prescribe the indicated medications and procedures, and to implement preventive strategies. Further infection and gangrene as a result of vascular insufficiency are continuing complications that always must be considered as a part of management strategies.

Other Skin Conditions

Other skin conditions include various forms of neoplasms, or tumors, such as fibroma and other cysts. They may require surgical removal if symptoms are present and usually are benign. Malignant neoplasms, such as melanoma, also can be present on the feet and require prompt and appropriate treatment. Other conditions include psoriasis and skin manifestations of diabetes, such as diabetic dermopathy (shin spots), necrobiosis lipoidica diabeticorum (fatty skin changes), and bullous diabeticorum (blisters).

For individuals with diabetes or other conditions that produce a sensory or arterial involvement, it is important to note the symptoms and findings, identified by Medicare, that permit the patient to qualify for some components of primary foot care (see Appendix). Medicare also provides coverage for the evaluation and management of an individual who has diabetes with diabetic sensory neuropathy that results in a loss of protective sensation as well as coverage for therapeutic shoes with customized multidensity insoles for at-risk individuals with diabetes (see Appendix).

TOENAIL PROBLEMS IN THE LONG-TERM CARE RESIDENT

Chief nail complaints usually relate to pain, thickness, hardness, and the inability to care for one's own toenails. These problems are magnified by poor eyesight, obesity, and the inability to bend. The normal toenail is somewhat thin and translucent, has a fresh pinkish color beneath the toenail, and has a slight medial to lateral curvature. However, toenails generally are hard and thickened in older adults, largely as a result of years of repetitive injury and a decreasing vascular supply to the nail bed. Among the causes of geriatric toenail pathology are trauma; infectious dermatoses; and degenerative diseases, such as arteriosclerosis, diabetes, and arthritis.

LTC staff should be aware that the older adult also might demonstrate anonychia (absence of a nail), macronychia (an enlarged nail), and micronychia (a small nail). These conditions usually are asymptomatic but should be documented for the individual's record.

Nail Plate

Thickening of the nail plate in the older adult is associated with aging; nutritional disturbances; repetitive trauma; inflammation; local infection; various infectious diseases, such as syphilis; and various degenerative diseases, such as arteriosclerosis. The nail will appear thickened or hypertrophic (onychauxis) and discolored. When thickening is accompanied by excessive hypertrophic deformity, onychogryphosis, or ram's horn nail (see Figure 3), is evident. Onychauxis that is left untreated will become onychogryphosis. Callus in the nail grooves (onychophosis) also may be present, and pain (onychalgia) is reported when touched, even by the upper part of the shoe or bed sheets. Subungual debris, subungual hyperkeratosis, and fungal infection (onychomycosis) may accompany this change in the nail plate. Periodic debridement is essential to provide relief of pain and reduce the potential for other complications, such as bacterial infection or ulceration.

A sudden traumatic blow or injury to the nail can result in a subungual hemorrhage (onychophyma, or bleeding under the toenail), followed by hematoma (dry collection of blood). Pain is significant from the hematoma. Bleeding usually can be seen through the translucent nail plate (Figure 12). A small hole may be drilled through the nail plate to permit the blood to escape, immediately relieving pain. X-rays should be taken to rule out a fracture of the bone. Thickening (onychauxis) may follow any acute injury to the nail root (matrix). A severe injury to the matrix also may cause loss of the toenail. When the loosening begins at the matrix area, it is termed *onychomadesis*. When the loosening begins at the free edge of the nail, it is termed *onycholysis*. Either may occur, depending on where the hematoma is located under the nail plate. Beau's lines (transverse striations) may follow to identify an interruption of nail growth (Figure 13), but the injury is not severe enough to cause shedding (onychoptosis) of the toenail.

Onychophosis (callus in the nail groove) usually is the result of repetitive minor trauma to the nail plate or some external pressure. A deformity such as incurvated or involuted nail plate (onychodysplasia) is also usually present. Treatment consists of debridement; the use of emollients, such as 20% to 40% urea to moisten, soften, and

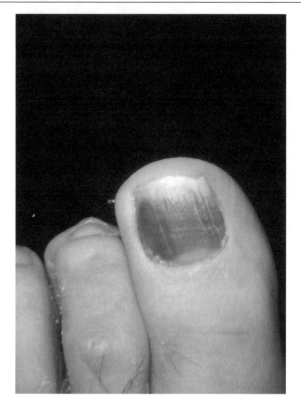

Figure 12. Subungual hematoma.

lubricate the hyperkeratosis (callus); thinning of the nail plate to permit flexibility; and removal of any external pressures. Where the nail deformity is severe or the nail lip is significantly hypertrophied, surgical revision should be considered.

Ingrown Toenail

Onychocryptosis (ingrown toenail) may occur when a fragment of the toenail pierces or penetrates the skin of the nail lip (ungualabia). It may result from improper self-treatment or external pressure. It may be accompanied by pain (onychalgia), inflammation (onychitis) of the nail and matrix areas (onychia), or the development of a secondary infection (paronychia) and periungual ulcerative granulation tissue. A subungual abscess also may appear initially. Conservative management depends on the clinical presentation. Excision of the offending

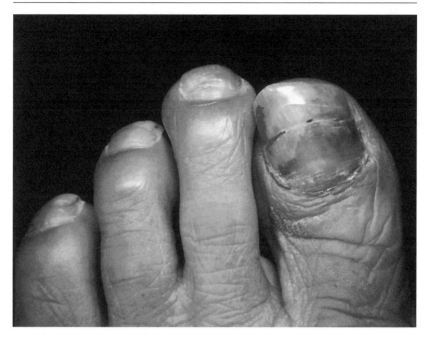

Figure 13. Transverse striation indicating interruption of nail growth (Beau's line).

portion of the toenail followed by mild compresses and a topical antibiotic should reduce the pain and inflammation. With infection, incision, drainage, and application of antibiotics are indicated. Total treatment can become complicated with a thickened or hypertrophied nail plate, such as involution (onychodysplasia). An ingrown toenail can become serious in the presence of systemic diseases, such as diabetes or arteriosclerosis, that compromise the circulatory and sensory systems. Neglect by the individual in these circumstances can result in a severe infection and the potential for necrosis or gangrene and possible amputation. When the condition does not respond to conservative measures or becomes ongoing, surgical excision and cautery of the granulation tissue of a portion of the nail and matrix may be considered to manage the condition and prevent further infection.

Subungual Heloma

Pinpoint pressure on the nail bed may result in a subungual heloma (corn). A bony tumor such as a subungual exostosis, spur, or a tumor formed from cartilage cells (chondroma) must be ruled out with imaging (X-ray) procedures. A deformity and hypertrophy of the superior, tufted end of the distal phalanx also is an etiologic factor that is demonstrable by X-ray. The corn appears as a dark spot beneath the nail plate. The potential of a cancerous tumor (subungual melanoma) always must be considered because of a similar clinical appearance and must be ruled out before any treatment can be instituted. Management consists of debriding of the lesion, thinning of the nail plate, and reducing pressure. With the presence of bony hypertrophy, surgical removal also must be considered.

Allergic Reactions

Allergic reactions in the toenails may be due to primary irritants, such as bacteria and fungi, or to repeated exposures to secondary irritants such as nail polish, polish removers, or shoe dyes. Inflammation (onychia) usually is present and is followed by a separation of the toenail from the nail bed, starting at the free edge (onycholysis). Degeneration of the nail plate (onychexallis), painful degeneration with hypertrophy (onychophyma), splitting of the nail plate (onychoschizia), and cracking (onychoclasis) also may occur. Treatment should be directed toward eliminating the cause, followed with medication for both inflammation and infection as indicated. Topical steroids may be useful for short periods in ongoing cases.

Remember that diet plays an important role in all body structures. In poor nutritional states, the nails usually become thin and brittle and lose their luster. Shedding may occur, beginning in the matrix, or posterior area (onychomadesis). Other trophic changes can follow, including atrophy (onychatrophia), dryness (onychia sicca), softening (onychomalacia), malformation (onychodystrophy), longitudinal ridging (onychorrhexis), and hypertrophic onychodystrophy (trophic nail change).

Fungal Infections

Onychomycosis is a fungal infection of the nail that usually causes a severe disturbance of nail growth accompanied by local nail plate destruction. The fungal infection may begin at the free edge, under the nail, along the lateral sides of the nail, or on the top of the toenail, known as superficial white mycosis. A candida infection is another possibility. In the older adult with ongoing health conditions, ony-chomycosis can be incapacitating as a result of deformity and infection. Onychomycosis always remains as a focal point for reinfection, particularly involving the skin, due to contact with the fungal organism. These toenails may appear opaque, scaly, and hypertrophic. The areas of fungal infection may be granular and may cause the nail to separate from the bed. Color changes may appear white, yellow, or brown, and there may be a musty odor, particularly when the diseased segment of the nail is removed. Treatment includes culture, potassium hydroxide (KOH) solution, mechanical debridement, dermabrasion, chemical debridement, and the use of antifungal agents; treatment may be topical, systemic, or a combination of multiple modalities. Onychomycosis in the older adult should be considered an ongoing health condition or infection and may require long-term management rather than cure. Antibiotics may be needed in the presence of bacterial infection. With ongoing health conditions such as diabetes and arteriosclerosis, the potential for complications is greater. Various neoplasms, or tumors, such as periungual verruca and melanoma, may affect the nail area. Therapy depends on the cause.

Other Conditions

Psoriatic nails usually are opaque and lose their luster. Loosening of the nails, debris, retarded growth, and Beau's lines are common. Inflammation is the classic diagnostic sign that a problem exists. Ongoing eczema usually produces a disturbed growth pattern and a marked nail distortion. Long-standing endocrine disturbances, such as thyroid disease, may cause atrophy of the nail plate and surrounding tissue but with repetitive trauma can demonstrate hypertrophic changes (continuing friction causes inflammation, increased cell growth, and friction). Diabetes may lead to diabetic onychopathy, hypertrophic onychodystrophy, and splinter hemorrhages under the nail plate. In the individual with diabetes, nail pathology can become serious quickly and may require hospitalization for management.

Restrictions of the blood supply to the toenail may produce atrophy and widening of the cuticle or hypertrophy of the eponychium (pterygium). When the eponychium hypertrophies and enlarges along the edge of the toenail, pain can be pronounced. Organic vascular diseases such as arteriosclerosis and Buerger's disease usually produce local ischemia and retarded linear growth. Splitting, brittleness, and overgrowth usually are present.

The nails of the individual with arthritis usually are dry and brittle. Toenails usually become inflamed and separated in the early stages and demonstrate hypertrophy in the later stages. It is important to remember that in the older adult, multiple ongoing health conditions usually are present and the clinical presentations may be varied and mixed and not conform to what might be considered a usual clinical presentation.

CONCLUSION

The skin and toenails are the easiest parts of the foot to observe. Older adults will have a variety of common skin and nail problems; those described in this chapter are but a few. Many of these can be managed easily with appropriate care, cleanliness, continuing surveillance, assessment, and professional care. In addition to being important for the comfort of the individual, skin and toenail conditions are significant because they are symptomatic of serious health problems.

CHAPTER FOUR

Identifying and Caring for Musculoskeletal Problems in the Long-Term Care Resident

"When your feet hurt, you hurt all over." This often-quoted adage probably originated because an elderly gentleman's feet hurt so badly that when he walked, he shifted his weight, walked abnormally, and thereby caused other joints to hurt. Although this may not be a true story, it is true that painful feet can cause pain elsewhere in the body. These foot problems in the older adult often are due to arthritis, partial dislocations, deformities associated with aging and diseases, and other mechanical (biomechanical and pathomechanical) disorders that affect the feet of older adults.

Movement is accomplished by the force of muscles and their tendons acting on bone of the body. Mechanical disorders occur when either the muscles or the bones are impaired, either structurally or functionally; therefore, they are termed *musculoskeletal disorders*. The following discussion examines the most common musculoskeletal problems of the foot and the procedures and principles in caring for them, including prevention.

COMMON MUSCULOSKELETAL PROBLEMS OF THE FOOT

As most things grow older, they tend to wear out and break down. This is true of automobiles and other machines with moving parts. It also is true of the human body. Years of use and abuse take their toll. Probably no area is affected more than the human foot, as a result of stress, disease, and a host of related environmental factors. The human foot was not designed to walk on hard, flat surfaces or to be exposed to the excessive stress of modern society. It has been estimated that a 65-year-old person has walked thousands of miles during his or her lifetime, a figure that the most well-constructed automobile, with interchangeable parts, cannot match. During the course of a lifetime, many changes occur, including wearing out of joints and loss of soft tissue. These changes affect not only the local area in which they occur but also other joints and areas that have to function with the affected joints. These changes in turn cause changes in posture, balance, and gait, as well as increase the risk for falling and limit mobility and may contribute to other musculoskeletal problems. These changes may affect the level of independent activity and daily life.

Musculoskeletal problems reveal themselves in many ways. Some of the symptoms and clinical findings include pain, gait change, difficulty in walking, changes in the shape and function of the foot, and the presence of foot deformities. Patients may report these as bumps, painful spurs, thickened skin, color changes, and crooked toes. Probably the most commonly reported source of discomfort and pain is the development of hyperkeratotic lesions, such as corns and calluses. Many people still consider these problems as primarily skin conditions and consequently apply various forms of topical preparations in an attempt to remove them. In fact, the use of commercial products that contain acid usually do more harm than good, and their use in individuals with ongoing systemic diseases, such as diabetes and peripheral arterial disease, is contraindicated and may cause ulceration, serious infection, and the potential for hospitalization and limb loss.

As pressure is applied to the skin, inflammation results, causing the upper layer of the skin to produce more cells as a protective response. With continuing pressure, skin cells continue to be produced, causing a thickening of the outer layer of the skin over the pressure point. The initial deformity, exaggerated by external pressure from inappropriate footwear, increases the inflammation, resulting in discomfort and pain. It is the underlying deformity or musculoskeletal change that is the primary cause in most individuals. Sidebar 1 lists the musculoskeletal changes that most often are identified with the older long-term care (LTC) resident.

Hammertoes

In older adults, the type of bony prominence that is seen most often is a condition called hammertoes. In a hammertoe, the toe joint contracts (hammers) or curves upward in the middle, subjecting the toe to external or shoe pressure and causes the formation of a hyperkeratotic lesion, such as a heloma, or corn. The development of hammertoes is associated with mechanical changes of the foot, tendon contractures, diseases such as rheumatoid arthritis and degen-

---

Musculoskeletal Changes of the Foot that Often Affect Older Long-Term Care Residents

- Gradual change in shape or size of the foot
- Soft tissue atrophy
- A sudden and painless change in foot shape with swelling and no history of trauma
- Cavus feet with claw toe
- Drop foot
- "Rocker bottom foot" or Charcot's foot
- Neuropathic arthropathy
- Elevated plantar pressure
- Decreased muscle strength
- Decreased ranges of motion
- Multiple foot deformities
- Limited joint mobility
- Hyperkeratosis (callus or corn)
- Abnormal foot pressure and subsequent ulceration
- Structural abnormalities or foot deformities:

Digiti flexus (hammertoes)	Tailor's bunion
	Plantar fasciitis
Claw toes	Myositis
Digital rotational deformities	Spur formation
	Calcaneal spurs
Prominent meta-tarsal heads	Enthesopathy
	Hyperostosis
Prolapsed meta-tarsal heads	Exostosis
	Bursitis
Atrophy of plan-tar fat pad	Periostitis
	Fibrositis
Plantar fat pad displacement	Decalcification
	Stress fractures
Plantar imbalance	Tendonitis
	Tenosynovitis
Foot muscle atrophy	Metatarsalgia
	Joint swelling
Hallux valgus	Haglund's
Hallux abducto valgus	deformity
	Neuritis
Hallux limitus	Entrapment
Hallux rigidus	syndrome
Morton's	Neuroma
syndrome	Sesamoid erosion

Sidebar 1

(continued)

Sidebar 1. *(continued)*

Sesamoid	Pes cavus
displacement	Equinus
Tendo-Achilles	Pes planus
contracture	Pes valgo planus
Digital	Residuals of
amputation	arthritis (de-
Partial foot	generative,
amputation	rheumatoid,
Charcot's joints	and gouty)
Phalangeal	Biomechanical
reabsorption	and patho-
Functional	mechanical
abnormalities	variations

erative arthritis, atrophy or wasting of the smaller intrinsic or internal muscles of the foot, and changes in foot function and shape as a result of the sum of life's activities.

One mechanical cause of hammertoes is the contracting of the tendons on the dorsum, or top, of the foot, which exerts a pull on the toe. If the toe is not in proper alignment, then the tendon will pull the toe abnormally and cause it to curve upward. There are a variety of hammertoes because there are two joints in each of the four lesser toes. Each may demonstrate some deformity, depending on external or shoe pressure, or gait changes. With continuing pressure, hyperkeratosis may form what can, in turn, lead to ulceration, infection, and additional complications, depending on the degree of peripheral arterial disease present (Figure 14). Continuing assessment and surveillance are essential in the presence of diabetes, arteriosclerosis, and a loss of protective sensation.

Osteoarthritis

Other musculoskeletal problems that often are seen in older adults are caused by osteoarthritis, or degenerative joint disease. This condition affects almost all older adults because, in this form of arthritis, the joints wear out from use, abuse, and repetitive trauma. The cartilage between the bones and on the joint surfaces begins to erode, causing bone to rub against bone, which causes pain. The erosion of cartilage also reduces the shock-absorbing quality of the joint and increases inflammation and limits motion. Some people claim that they can forecast the weather mainly by the pain that they experience before a change in humidity or barometric pressure. Radiographs (X-rays) demonstrate areas of bone spur formation around the joints and a narrowing of the spaces between the joints. There also may be some ob-

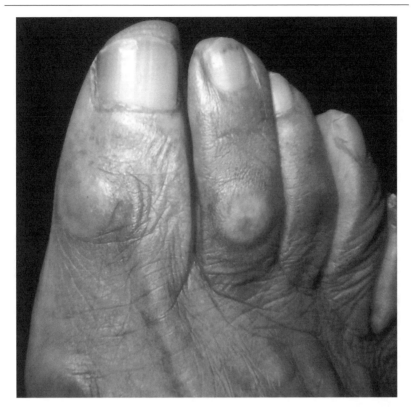

Figure 14. Hammertoes with heloma, early subkeratotic hematoma, and early pressure ulcer.

servable thickening of the joints of the fingers and the toes. Most individuals with degenerative joint disease experience stiffness in the morning, which decreases as the day progresses and the joints are exercised. Sidebar 2 lists the most common clinical findings that are associated with degenerative joint disease.

Rheumatoid Arthritis

Another type of arthritis that often is seen in the LTC resident is rheumatoid arthritis, a disease that affects connective tissue. It differs from degenerative joint disease in that the joints do not merely wear out from long-term use but instead eventually are destroyed completely. Rheumatoid arthritis is one of many collagen (connec-

Most Common Clinical Findings Associated with Degenerative Joint Disease

- Plantar fasciitis
- Spur formation
- Periostitis
- Decalcification
- Stress fractures
- Tendonitis
- Tenosynovitis
- Residual deformities
- Pes planus
- Pronation
- Pes cavus
- Hallux valgus
- Hallux varus
- Hallux limitus
- Hallux rigidus
- Hallux flexus
- Digiti flexus (hammertoes)
- Rotational digital deformities
- Digiti quinti varus
- Overriding toes
- Underriding toes
- Prolapsed metatarsals
- Joint swelling
- Increased pain
- Limitation of motion
- Splay foot
- Reduced ambulatory status

Sidebar 2

tive tissue) diseases that are believed to have an autoimmune factor in their cause.

Rheumatoid arthritis causes dislocation of joints, usually laterally; joint fusions; and bunion, or hallux valgus, formation. Many musculoskeletal conditions can be caused by rheumatoid arthritis, including hammertoes, bowstring tendons, complete disappearance of toe bones, and other joint deformities (Figure 15). X-rays of individuals with rheumatoid arthritis demonstrate destroyed joints, loss of calcium in the bones, brittleness of bones, and dislocated and misaligned toes. Sidebar 3 lists some of the residuals of rheumatoid arthritis.

Bunions

The term *bunion* is used to describe a variety of diagnostic categories with an associated enlargement of the medial, or inner, side of the great toe joint. Enlargement usually is accompanied by swelling, bony enlargement, inflammation, limitation of motion, and pain. In most cases, the bone actually is normal in consistency but with joint deformity. The first metatarsal usually is forced in an inward direction. The great toe is forced in a lateral, or outward, direction. This deviation moves the great toe toward the second toe, and overlapping is common when the deformity is significant. Shoes do not cause bunions in the LTC resident. They are caused by a variety of anatomic variations, arthritic changes, soft tissue contractures, inflammation, and biomechanical and pathomechanical alterations. Joint hypermobility and a congenital shortening of the first metatarsal bone both are examples of such alterations.

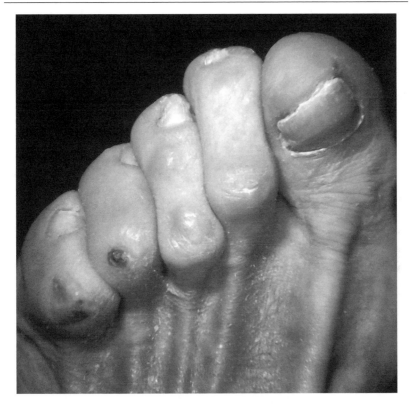

Figure 15. Rheumatoid arthritis with hammertoes and bowstring tendons.

Metatarsalgia

Another musculoskeletal disorder involves pain in the ball of the foot, usually diagnosed as metatarsalgia. Individuals who are ambulatory usually complain of a dull ache or pain or a burning sensation in the ball of the foot. In the older adult, the soft tissue fat pad that absorbs shock and disperses pressure usually atrophies and literally disappears. The metatarsal head usually can be palpated, or felt, just beneath the skin. This area of the foot now has only fascia and tendons to absorb shock and pressure. In addition, joint changes as a result of degenerative joint diseases increase the deformity and add prominence to the metatarsal heads themselves. It is the irritation and inflammation that cause pain and may increase soft tissue swelling. In

Some Residuals of Rheumatoid Arthritis	
• Hallux limitus	• Tendon displacement
• Hallux rigidus	• Ganglions
• Hallux valgus	• Rigid pronation
• Hallux abducto valgus	• Subcalcaneal bursitis
• Cystic erosion	• Retrocalcaneal bursitis
• Sesamoid erosion	• Retro-Achilles bursitis
• Sesamoid displacement	• Calcaneal ossifying enthesopathy (spur)
• Metatarsophalangeal subluxation	• Prolapsed metatarsal heads
• Metatarsophalangeal dislocation	• Atrophy and/or displacement of the plantar fat pad
• Interphlangeal subluxation	• Digiti quinti varus
• Interphalangeal dislocation	• Tailor's bunion
• Digiti flexus (hammertoe)	• Early-morning stiffness
• Ankylosis (fused joints)	• Pain
• Phalangeal reabsorption	• Fibrosis
• Talo-navicular arthritis	• Contracture
• Extensor tenosynovitis	• Deformity
• Rheumatoid nodules	• Impairment
• Bowstring extensor tendons	• Reduction of ambulation

Sidebar 3

addition, the bursa that surround each joint may become inflamed, resulting in anterior metatarsal bursitis.

Bunionettes

On the lateral side, or outside, of the foot, in the area posterior to, or behind, the fifth toe, swelling and deformity may occur; this is known as a bunionette, or tailor's bunion. There usually is some lateral, or outward, displacement of the fifth metatarsal and an inward, or medial, displacement of the fifth toe, with some enlargement of the fifth metatarsal phalangeal joint. In the older adult, degenerative joint changes also usually are present. Hyperkeratosis may form with pressure.

Other Disorders of the Hallux

Other disorders that limit motion at the hallux, or great toe joint, are hallux limitus and hallux rigidus. Both represent a monoarticular, or single-joint, arthritis that is degenerative in nature. There is an enlargement of the first metatarsal head with spur formation on the dorsum, or top, of the joint. Similar spur formation may be noted on the superior, or upper, surface of the base of the proximal phalanx of the great toe. Motion creates inflammation, and the spur formation limits motion. Hallux limitus permits limited motion. With hallux rigidus, the spurs are severe and there is almost no motion at the joint. X-rays, especially the lateral view of the joint, will identify the pathology clearly. When the joint bends in walking, there is inflammation and pain. Restriction of motion reduces the inflammation and reduces pain.

CARING FOR MUSCULOSKELETAL DISORDERS

As a part of the patient assessment, musculoskeletal strength of the dorsiflexors, plantarflexors, invertors, and evertors should be noted. The presence of atrophy, particularly involving the foot and the leg, is important. Gait evaluation should include foot type, heel-to-toe pattern, eversion, inversion, foot structural change, and ambulatory aids. Gait evaluation also should include shoe evaluation as to the type of shoe, fit, and size; shoe wear and patterns of wear; shoe lining wear; the presence of foreign bodies; the type of insoles; and orthoses.

Osteoarthritis

The management of degenerative joint disease for the LTC resident involves reducing pain and increasing motion to maintain ambulation. Treatment may include the use of physical modalities such as whirlpool, ultrasound, paraffin baths, and other forms of mild heat, which surround the inflamed joint. This seems to relax the muscles, relieve some of the joint pressure, and allow for smoother and less painful motion. Mild analgesics usually will help to control moderate discomfort. Exercise programs also are important to help strengthen muscles and maintain mobility. Orthotics, bracing, and mobility aids can be used to assist in ambulation and support inflamed joints. Surgical consideration may be indicated and can include joint replacement and joint fusion. Additional management considerations include

- Radiographs (weight and non–weight bearing)
- Nonsteroidal anti-inflammatory drugs
- Local steroid injections
- Superficial and deep heat (with caution)
- Muscle stimulation, contractile currents
- Transcutaneous electrical nerve stimulation

- Shoe last changes
- Internal shoe modifications
- External shoe modifications
- Special last and/or extra-depth shoes
- Custom-molded shoes
- Orthoses for weight diffusion, dispersion, support, and dynamics

Rheumatoid Arthritis

For the older adult with rheumatoid arthritis, the focus of care is management rather than cure, which is true for most ongoing health conditions. Treatment is concerned with symptoms, that is, controlling the pain, restoring the maximum function possible, and maintaining that function once restored. Methods include managing deformities and slowing their progression with braces, shoes, and orthoses as well as physical modalities and procedures, such as whirlpool, ultrasound, and daily exercise programs. Surgical joint revision and the replacement of joints have been a great help to individuals with rheumatoid arthritis. The decision to attempt these procedures in LTC residents is based on judgment, symptoms, and the quality of life to be maintained, as is true after any surgical intervention.

Biomechanical and Pathomechanical Deformities

The biomechanical and pathomechanical deformities of the feet and related structures usually can be managed in a conservative manner. Pes planus and pes valgo planus, referred to as flat feet and pronation if symptomatic, usually requires the use of radiographs for an appropriate diagnosis, followed by some form of orthosis and/or shoe modification. Again, the determination of care should be based on the quality of life, ambulatory status, activities of daily living (e.g., grooming, bathing), instrumental activities of daily living (e.g., shopping, housekeeping, transportation), and the relationship of management to the functional needs of the individual.

Bunions

Management of bunions in the LTC resident needs to consider pain, the ambulatory status of the individual, the projected outcome, potential complications in the older adult, and the functional needs of the individual. Radiographs should be taken initially to determine the extent of anatomic and pathological change. Special shoes, orthotics, physical modalities, exercise, and surgical revision all are considerations and are based on the individual's needs. Joint stabilization with an orthodigital device also is an early consideration. Observation for signs of inflammation, excessive pressure, and ulceration are important elements of the continuing surveillance of foot deformities.

Metatarsalgia

The use of physical modalities, such as mild heat and ultrasound, along with shoe modification and orthotics that act as soft tissue replacement usually permit pressure and pain to be reduced, weight to be redistributed, and the individual to ambulate in comfort. Local steroid injections also may be indicated in the acute phase. Radiographs are indicated to rule out the possibility of a stress fracture.

Bunionettes

Management of bunionettes from a conservative point of view includes pressure reduction and shoe modification. For the LTC resident, surgical revision may be indicated, as based on the symptoms and ambulatory needs of the individual.

Other Disorders of the Hallux

Conservative management of other disorders of the hallux includes the use of physical modalities; local steroid injections; and placement of a steel shank extension under the great toe joint, between the insole and the outsole, to limit motion and restrict bending. Padding, use of a low-vamp shoe, and reduction of pressure by changing the shoe last can relieve pressure around the joint. For example, a Velcro strap can be adjusted more easily than shoelaces. Surgical revision of the joint and/or joint replacement is an additional option and should be considered if indicated.

Combinations of Disorders

In the high-arched, or cavus, foot, it is not uncommon to see tyloma (calluses), heloma (corns), hallux valgus (bunion), and hammertoes all in the same patient. With degenerative changes, atrophy and displacement of the plantar metatarsal fat pad, contractures, and the residuals of arthritis, discomfort and pain may be significant. There usually is some degree of metatarsal head prolapse, clinically, and individuals complain that it feels like they are walking on the bones of their feet. In a sense, they are. Appropriate functional orthotics that are multidensity in composition usually provide comfort in a manner similar to those used in extra-depth shoes for at-risk patients, such as those with diabetes. Orthosis and shoe modification are a reasonable conservative approach to management for the LTC resident.

Occasionally, an individual will complain of a sharp, burning pain between two toes that occurs while walking and usually stops when there is no weight or pressure on the foot. The pain clearly is relieved when the individual removes his or her shoes. The cause may be an enlarged and inflamed interdigital nerve, which is associated directly with compression in the metatarsal head area and other biomechanical changes. The pain usually is associated with the lateral four metatarsal heads; with chronic inflammation, there is an associated enlargement of the neural sheath. Management approaches include radiographs; magnetic resonance imaging; physical modalities; a wider shoe last; padding and/or orthotics to change the intermetatarsal head position; local steroid injection; and, when conservative measures fail, surgical excision.

Calcaneal spurs with heel pain and associated plantar fasciitis are other manifestations of musculoskeletal problems. In the older adult, the shock-absorbing fat pad that protects the heel is lost. Also, the ligaments are relaxed and weakened, stretched, and allow positional changes in the foot. The stress causes a calcification of the attachment of the plantar fascia, usually at the medial, or inner, tuberosity. A residual bursitis also may be noted. Pain may be associated with plantar fasciitis, bursitis, calcaneal spur, or periostitis or may be a combination of one or more of these clinical conditions. The symptoms usually indicate that pain initially occurs on first standing and bearing weight and walking. Symptoms gradually lessen and then return after the individual sits and then begins to walk again. It is the initial stress on the plantar fascia that precipitates the initial inflammation and pain. Management includes the use of physical modalities, such as ultrasound with phonophoresis, local steroid injections, exercise, heel cups, night splints, shoe modification and padding, and orthotics. For the older LTC resident with these conditions, conservative management usually relieves the symptoms and permits the individual to walk without pain.

Other Considerations

In recognizing problems that are associated with musculoskeletal disorders, there are mechanical factors that need to be considered:

- Body mass
- Gait
- Ambulatory speed
- Tissue trauma
- Weight diffusion
- Weight dispersion
- Pathomechanics (defined as structural change in relation to function)
- Biomechanics (defined as forces that change and affect the foot in relation to function)
- Imbalance (defined as the inability to adapt to alterations of stress)
- Various forms of stress:

  Force (alteration in physical condition, either shape or position)

  Compression stress (one force moves toward another)

  Tensile stress (a pulling away of one part against another)

Shearing stress (a sliding of one part on the other)

Friction (the force needed to overcome resistance and usually associated with a sheering stress)

Elasticity (weight diffusion and weight dispersion)

Fluid pressure (soft tissue adaptation and conformity to stress)

In addition, the use of orthotics in the LTC resident must be based on the individual's ability to use the modification and willingness of staff to assist the individual. Shoes and orthotics must be used in concert, and, in some cases, the orthotic must be cemented into the shoe. Orthotics protect, restore, or improve function of moveable parts of the body with orthopedic appliances or an apparatus that supports, aligns, prevents, or corrects deformities. Foot orthotics may or may not include a shoe and/or any modifications or transfers that are necessary to make the orthotic functional and effective. They are fabricated to meet the specific needs of the individual.

Care entails prevention. Preventing musculoskeletal problems in the older LTC resident requires early recognition, comprehensive management based on the individual's needs, and proper selection of footwear and ambulatory aids.

CONCLUSION

As muscles age, they may atrophy and weaken. These weaknesses affect not only the immediate local area but also every associated bone, joint, and muscle, thereby leading to painful deformities. All of these clinical conditions have one common thread: When untreated, they cause the individual to walk and live in pain and distress. Older adults seem to lose their enthusiasm when they become bedridden or helpless because of foot problems. Foot pain in the older adult reduces the physical and mental aspects of quality of life as well as mobility, which limits independent living.

CHAPTER FIVE

Complications Involving the Vascular, Neurological, and Endocrine Systems

S ome of the most disabling conditions and complications that can affect the feet and lower extremities of the long-term care (LTC) resident are peripheral vascular disease, neurological conditions, and the related changes of the diabetic foot. It is of paramount importance for the staff of all LTC programs and facilities to be aware of the presence of the initial signs, symptoms, and complications that modify the arterial vascular flow in the extremities, present with other vascular symptoms, create insensitivity of the lower extremities, and impair functional activity as a result of neurological changes. Many of the most common diseases of older adults—cognitive impairment, diabetes, heart failure, cerebrovascular accidents, hypertension, arthritis,

Alzheimer's disease, dementia, depression, allergies, and anemia—usually present with foot symptoms and related complications.

PERIPHERAL VASCULAR DISEASE

Vascular diseases are conditions that affect the blood vessels. Many forms of peripheral vascular diseases can be identified in the legs and the feet of older adults, in particular in those who reside in LTC programs and facilities. It is important to recognize the symptoms and signs of these conditions, assess their clinical significance, and prevent complications through early consultation and management. In general, peripheral vascular diseases involve the arterial, venous, and lymphatic systems.

The most common forms of peripheral arterial disease (PAD) or lower extremity arterial disease include arteriosclerosis, atherosclerosis, Raynaud's disease, Raynaud's phenomenon, arterial thrombosis, arterial embolism, thromboangiitis obliterans (Buerger's disease), bruits, and abdominal aortic aneurysm. The most common venous diseases that present in the legs and the feet are deep venous thrombosis, deep thrombophlebitis, superficial thrombophlebitis, venous insufficiency, venous stasis, and varicosities. The most common lymphatic problems, both pitting and nonpitting, are those that are associated with edema and swelling of the feet and legs: congenital and secondary lymphatic disorders and disorders secondary to other systemic and local conditions such as arterial vasospasm, Paget's disease, congestive heart failure, dependency of the lower extremity, postphlebitic syndrome, and varicosities. Inasmuch as the majority of peripheral vascular diseases are diagnosed before or at admission, management represents a team approach that is directed by the attending or admitting physician in concert with the consulting and facility staff.

Arteriosclerosis usually refers to a disease that is characterized by a thickening of the muscular layers of the arterial system and a loss of elasticity and may include calcification. Atherosclerosis is similar in the loss of elasticity and narrowing of the arteries but is attributed to fatty deposits within the interior wall of the vessel. The symptoms can be similar to those of arteriosclerosis because both diseases decrease blood flow. It also is important to recognize the acute symptoms of

PAD and lower extremity arterial disease—coldness, numbness, and thrombosis—from those of chronic arterial disease—burning pain that usually is relieved by rest and aggravated by standing. The acute phase can result in amputation and may be life threatening if not recognized and managed early in an individual's care.

PERIPHERAL ARTERIAL DISEASE

PAD and/or peripheral arteriosclerotic disease of the lower extremities produces a narrowing of the blood vessels and restriction of blood flow to the legs and the feet. Both atherosclerosis and calcification of vessels can be demonstrated in the older adult. Risk factors for development of PAD include age more than 65 years, history of smoking, Buerger's disease, Raynaud's disease or syndrome, high blood pressure, high cholesterol, and diabetes. People who have arteriosclerosis, or hardening of the arteries, of the heart and the brain are more likely to develop PAD, which can be a risk factor for heart attack or stroke. Some of the primary complications include inadequate soft tissue perfusion, nonhealing wounds, infection, ulceration, tissue loss, and the potential for amputation. These problems increase the potential for LTC admission and significantly reduce the quality of life for residents of LTC facilities.

The most common symptoms include coldness; pain; achy, tired sensation in the feet and the legs; and intermittent claudication, cramping, or aching of the feet, calves, thighs, or buttocks when walking that usually is relieved by rest. For LTC residents with decreased ambulation, intermittent claudication may not be reported as a significant complaint. There are other causes of intermittent claudication-like symptoms: arthritis of the hips, restless legs syndrome, peripheral neuropathies, spinal stenosis, prolapsed or compressed intervertebral disc, osteoporosis, and altered foot biomechanics and pathomechanics. Taking of medical, surgical, and social history is important. In addition, the associated medical, nutritional, and ambulatory status of the individual is important. Sidebar 4 lists the primary symptoms of peripheral arterial impairment. Sidebar 5 lists the primary clinical findings that are associated with peripheral arterial impairment.

It is important to stratify the level of risk for complications for patients with peripheral arterial insufficiency or disease (see Appen-

Primary Symptoms of Peripheral Arterial Impairment
• Fatigue
• Cramps
• Pain
• Intermittent claudication (calf pain)
• Muscle or limb weakness with use
• Ischemia
• Temperature changes (coolness)
• Night or foot pain in resting limb that is relieved by standing or placing the legs over the side of the bed
• Paresthesia (numbness and/or tingling)
• Color changes: rubor (red) or cyanosis (blue)
• Night cramps
• Burning
• Edema (swelling)
• Poor healing
• Pallor
• Blebs (blisters)
• Ulceration
• Necrosis and gangrene
• Venous swelling and/or varicosities

Sidebar 4

dix [Risk Category–Vascular] for an example of such a clinical classification). The clinical procedures that are used to evaluate the vascular status of older adults, particularly those in LTC facilities, are an important factor in preventing arteriosclerotic ulceration, infection, necrosis, gangrene, and loss of life; they include a visual inspection of the lower extremity and palpation of pulses, including pedal, popliteal, and femoral.

Other findings include skin color, skin integrity, evidence of pallor on elevation, rubor on dependency, with color returning to normal above the 20-second delay after elevation. Testing includes the use of a Doppler to assess pulses if they are not patent. Oscillometric studies also will demonstrate a decreased response with arterial insufficiency. These results may be modified by the presence of edema, induration, and vessel calcification. A radiometer can determine skin temperature and also can determine "hot spots," which may be early indicators of infection and ulceration.

Testing may be invasive (arteriography with intravenous contrast), less invasive (digital subtraction angiography), or noninvasive (magnetic resonance imaging, computed tomographic arteriography, and Doppler imaging) and may include anatomic imaging. Other noninvasive procedures include the oscillometer index, Duplex ultrasonography, and measurement of the ankle brachial index (ABI; dividing the brachial artery pressure into the systolic pressure of some of the pedal arteries) using these measurements:

An index of 0.09–1.2 is considered a normal resting index

Normal ABI >0.9

Mild ABI $< 0.9 - 0.75$

Moderate ABI $< 0.75 - 0.4$

Ischemic rest pain < 0.5

Threatened limb < 0.15

Tissue loss < 0.5

Treatable ischemia < -0.15

Other studies that may be used include segmental pressure measurement, plethysmographic waveform analysis (pulse volume recording), skin perfusion pressure, laser Doppler pressure, color Doppler imaging and ultrasonography, transcutaneous oxygen content, cutaneous oximetry, and treadmill exercise testing (claudication time measurement). The use of specialized testing should be determined as indicated on the basis of the needs of the individual and with a concern for management outcomes and avoiding excessive stress for older adults. For older adults with diabetes, some of the signs and symptoms may be decreased as a result of neuropathy.

Management considerations include the following:

- Risk factor modification, such as smoking cessation, controlling hypertension, treating dyslipidemia, and

Primary Clinical Findings Associated with Peripheral Arterial Impairment

- Decreased or absent dorsalis pedis pulse
- Decreased or absent posterior tibial pulse
- Decreased or absent popliteal pulse
- Femoral pulse change
- Prolonged digital capillary reflux filling time (greater than 3–4 seconds)
- Edema
- Tissue loss
- Ulceration (ischemic, punched out, little bleeding, and pain)
- Superficial infections:
  Bacterial
  Mycotic
- Delayed venous filling time (exceeding 10 seconds)
- Soft tissue atrophy
- Trophic changes:
  Hair (decreased or absent)
  Skin color (rubor, dependent rubor)
  Skin texture:
    Thin, shiny, dystrophic, and parchment like
    Hair loss
  Xerosis (dryness)
  Fissures
  Maceration
  Pigmentary changes and skin discoloration: hemosiderin deposition
- Onychial changes:
  Onychopathy
  Onychorrhexis (can be caused by nutritional change)
  Onycholysis
  Onychomadesis
  Thickening with deformity
  Onychauxis
  Onychogryphosis
  Brittleness
  Onychodystrophy
  Onychodysplasia
  Onychophosis

Sidebar 5

(continued)

Sidebar 5. *(continued)*

> Onychomycosis
> Subungual keratosis
> Discoloration
> Subungual hematoma (splinter
>   hemorrhages)
> • Color change:
>   Cyanosis
>   Dependent rubor
>   Pallor
>   Erythema
> • Temperature changes (coldness or
>   decreased warmth)
> • Vascular bruits
> • Edema
> • Necrosis (localized and demarcated)
> • Gangrene
> • Possible associated phlebitis
> • Muscle wasting
> • Muscle fatigue
>   Atrophy of plantar fat pad

managing and controlling diabetes

• Prescribing pharmacologic agents such as antiplatelet drugs and other medications to decrease the frequency and the severity of intermittent claudication

• Exercise and rehabilitation, such as increased walking and treadmill use

• Appropriate foot care, including patient education, primary podiatric medicine, and appropriate footwear

• Surgical intervention as indicated, including lower extremity angioplasty, bypass surgery, and potential amputation.

NEUROLOGICAL CONDITIONS

Neurological diseases are conditions that affect the nervous system. Many forms of neurological conditions and diseases can be identified in the legs and the feet of older adults, in particular in those who reside in LTC programs and facilities. It is important to recognize the symptoms and signs of these conditions, assess their clinical significance, and prevent complications through early consultation and management. The primary symptoms of neurological impairments in older individuals include but are not limited to the signs listed in Sidebar 6.

For the most part, most of the neurological conditions that present in LTC residents are diagnosed before or at admission. Some of the primary diseases include amyotrophic lateral sclerosis, cerebral palsy, cerebrovascular accident or stroke, Guillain-Barré syndrome, herpes zoster, Huntington's chorea, lumbar disk disorders and spinal stenosis, multiple sclerosis, muscular dystrophy, Parkinson's disease, vitamin deficiencies, and the neuropathic symptoms that are associated with diabetes. Other related conditions include gait disorders, neuromuscular weakness, the neurological manifestations of rheumatologic disease, metabolic and endocrine disorders, trauma, entrapment, reflex sympathetic dystrophy, and chronic pain. The management of neurological conditions in the LTC facility requires a team approach under the direction of the admitting or attending physician in concert with the consulting and facility staff.

The most common neurological symptoms include gait changes that are associated with ambulatory dysfunction; reflex changes, including the patellar, Achilles, and superficial plantar; ankle clonus; diminished or a loss of the vibratory sense; weakness; sensory deficits; change in proprioception; pain or podalgia; changes in temperature perception; hyperesthesia or anesthesia; autonomic dysfunction; and a loss of protective sensation. A medical, surgical, social, and nutritional history as well as the ambulatory status of the patient also is important.

Primary Symptoms of Neurological Impairments in Older Individuals

- Sensory impairment:
  Burning
  Tingling
  Clawing sensations
  Paresthesia
- Pain (podalgia) and hyperactivity
- Two-point discrimination
- Motor changes:
  Weakness
  Foot drop
- Autonomic responses:
  Diminished sweating
  Hyperhidrosis
- Sensory deficits:
  Vibratory
  Proprioceptive
- Loss of protective sensation
- Changes in pain and temperature perception
- Hyperesthesia
- Diminished to absent deep tendon reflexes (Achilles and patellar)
- Superficial plantar reflex change
- Hypohidrosis with perfusion
- Dermopathy or pretibial lesions (shin spots)
- Thickened skin with calluses under high-pressure areas, demonstrating an intrinsic minus foot (marked digital contractures, metatarsal prolapse, prominent metatarsal heads, and plantar fat pad atrophy and displacement)
- Muscle atrophy
- Bowstring tendons
- Neurotrophic osteoarthropathy (Charcot's foot)
- Neurotrophic ulceration

Sidebar 6

DIABETIC FOOT CHANGES

Foot problems that are related to diabetes are focused to some degree on the vascular and neurological complications as well as musculoskeletal and dermatological complications and changes that are associated with aging. The majority of the clinical findings that have been discussed in the chapters that deal with skin, toenail, and musculoskeletal changes, as well as the sections in this chapter that deal with peripheral vascular and neurological changes apply, for the most part, to older adults with diabetes.

Amputation and foot ulceration are the most common consequences of diabetic neuropathy and a major cause of morbidity and disability in people with diabetes. Early recognition and management of independent risk factors can prevent or delay adverse outcomes. The risk for ulcers or amputations is increased in people who have had diabetes for more than 10 years; are male; have poor glucose control; or have cardiovascular, retinal, or renal complications. The following foot-related risk conditions are associated with an increased risk for amputation:

- Peripheral neuropathy with loss of protective sensation
- Altered biomechanics (in the presence of neuropathy)
- Evidence of increased pressure (erythema, hemorrhage under a callus)
- Fat pad atrophy and/or displacement
- Limited joint mobility
- Structural and bony deformity
- Peripheral vascular disease (decreased or absent pedal pulses)
- History of ulcers or amputation
- Severe nail pathology

Targeted patient education and appropriate footwear can reduce the risk for ulceration. Some of the other factors that contribute to the development of foot problems in the older adult with diabetes include but are not limited to the following:

- Degree of ambulation
- Gait change and/or ambulatory dysfunction
- Duration of any previous hospitalization
- Limitation of activity

- Previous social segregation or living alone

- Previous care

- Duration of diabetes (more than 10 years)

- Individual's adjustment to life and diabetes

- Polypharmacy

- History of alcohol and/or tobacco use

- Obesity

- Impaired vision

- Dementia

- Complications that are associated with other risk diseases, such as cardiovascular disease, renal disease, retinal disease, osteoarthritis, rheumatoid arthritis, gout, neurological diseases, and PAD

Sidebar 7 lists the most common symptoms and signs that are associated with the diabetic foot in the older adult.

The Appendix lists the Medicare criteria for assessment and stratification of a loss of protective sensation in individuals with diabetes as well as criteria to qualify for therapeutic shoes. In assessing older LTC residents who have diabetes and are ambulatory, it is important to eval-

Most Common Symptoms Associated with the Diabetic Foot in the Older Adult	
• Vascular impairment	• Necrosis
• Degenerative joint changes	• Gangrene
• Aging	• Pallor
• Neuropathy	• Absent or decrease of posterior tibial and dorsalis pedis pulses
• Dermopathy	
• Atrophy of soft tissue	
• Insensitivity	• Dependent rubor
• Paresthesia	• Delayed venous filling time
• Sensory impairment to pain and temperature	• Coolness of the skin
• Motor weakness	• Trophic changes
• Limited joint mobility and/or range of motion	• Numbness
	• Tingling
• Stress fractures	• Cramps
• Diminished or loss of Achilles and patellar reflexes	• Pain
	• Atrophy, displacement, or loss of the plantar metatarsal fat pad
• Decreased or absent vibratory sense (pallesthesia)	• Elevated plantar pressure
• Loss of proprioception	• Hyperkeratotic lesions
• Loss of protective sensation	• Tendon contractures
• Xerosis	• Neuroma
• Anhidrosis	• Neuritis
• Neurotrophic arthropathy	• Soft tissue inflammation Bursitis Tendonitis Fasciitis
• Neurotrophic ulcers	
• Disparity or gradual change in foot size and shape	• Ulceration
	• Foot drop
• Higher prevalence of infection	• Diabetic dermopathy (pretibial lesions [shin spots])

Sidebar 7

(continued)

Sidebar 7. *(continued)*

• Neurotrophic arthropathy Charcot's foot Rocker bottom foot	Osteolysis Deformities Osteoporosis Reabsorption
• Deformity (structural) Hallux valgus Hallux limitus, hallux rigidus Claw toes and/or hammertoes Tailor's bunion Spur formation Pes cavus Pes planus	• Pruritus • Cutaneous infections • Dehydration • Trophic changes • Fissures • Functional abnormalities • Footwear considerations:
• Radiographic	Type of shoe
• Thin trabecular patterns: Decalcification Joint position change Osteophytic formation	Last Fit and size Shoe wear patterns Shoe lining wear Insoles Orthoses Foreign bodies

uate the mechanical factors that contribute to the potential for ulcer formation, which are listed in Chapter 4 for musculoskeletal disorders.

The ulcerations that LTC residents usually have include arterial (PAD), venous, and diabetic, which are related to pressure. For the most part, diabetic and pressure ulcers have some similar etiologic concerns, including pressure, friction, shearing, and maceration (Figures 16 and 17). Similar associated etiologic factors include systemic diseases, poor nutrition, soft tissue atrophy, bony abnormalities, anemia, infection, edema, tumors, polycythemia vera, congestive heart failure, lymphedema, renal failure, hypothyroidism, related environmental factors, and trauma (mechanical, chemical, and thermal). Some of the assessment factors for stress ulcers include but are not limited to the following:

- Comorbidity

- Nutritional assessment

- Pain assessment

- Wound assessment

    Stage I: Nonblanchable erythema of intact skin (heralding lesion [reactive hyperemia])

    Stage II: Superficial, presents as an abrasion, blister, or shallow crater (partial skin loss) in epidermis and/or dermis

    Stage III: Full-thickness skin loss involving damage or necrosis of subcutaneous tissue; may extend to fascia

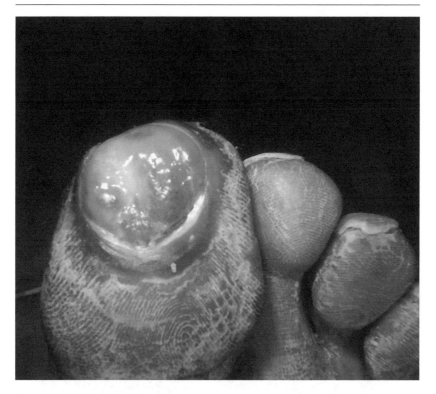

Figure 16. Diabetic ulcer.

Stage IV: Full thickness wounds with extensive destruction, tissue necrosis, or damage to muscle, bone, or supporting structures (sinus tracts, osteomyelitis, septic arthritis)

The management of pedal ulcers and wound care involves a wide range of medical and surgical options. Providing pressure reduction is important, as is the management of infection with appropriate antibiotics. Active wound care management may include surgical débridement with documentation of the duration of the ulcer or wound, size of the ulcer or wound, depth of the ulcer or wound, and the amount of necrotic tissue present. Treatment parameters encompass multiple factors that include but are not limited to the following:

- Mental status of the individual
- Mobility and ambulatory status of the individual

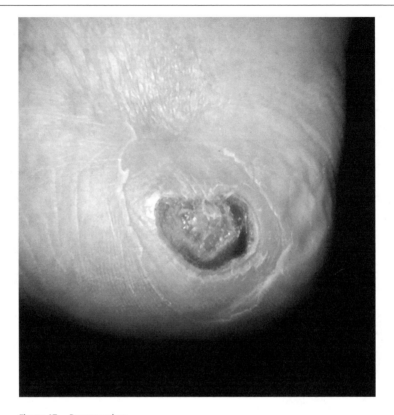

Figure 17. Pressure ulcer.

- Infection and antibiotic management
- Degree of tissue oxygenation
- Chronic pressure findings and management
- Arterial insufficiencies (PAD)
- Venous status and management
- Edema, including cause and management
- Type of dressing and management
- Presence of certain chronic conditions:

    Diabetes

    Uremia

    Chronic obstructive pulmonary disease

Malnutrition

Congestive heart failure

Anemia

Immune deficiency disorders

PAD

Chronic venous disease

Indurated edema

Management considerations usually include the relief of pressure, the control of infection, and appropriate debridement. The patient care and record documentation should include the specific signs and symptoms and other clinical data to support the diagnosis; other medical conditions; wound status; and the patient's response to treatment. The record of patient management also should include the medical diagnosis; the wound stage or the level/depth of the tissue debrided; the wound characteristics, such as diameter, color, and presence of exudates or necrotic tissue; the vascular status of the patient; the appropriate vascular and/or surgical evaluation; and the patient's specific goals and/or response to treatment. Appropriate review and consultation by the attending or admitting physician and the appropriate specialties should be used to manage the patient's condition to maintain the individual's quality of life.

CONCLUSION

Foot pain and diseases and disorders of the feet and their related structures in the older adult limit mobility and reduce the physical and mental aspects of the quality of life. For maintaining foot health, practitioners and staff must think comprehensively and recognize that team care must be an essential part of geriatrics, gerontology, and the management of chronic disease.

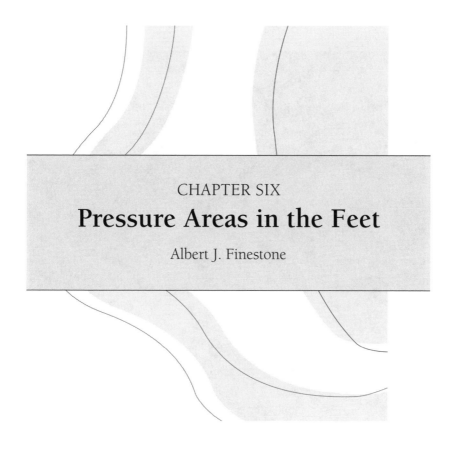

CHAPTER SIX

Pressure Areas in the Feet

Albert J. Finestone

A major challenge in long-term care (LTC) residents is avoidance of pressure ulcers in the lower extremities. An additional factor that must be considered is the revised Federal Regulation from the Centers for Medicare and Medicaid Services for pressure ulcer care in LTC facilities.[1] The new report considerably expands the guideline to state and federal surveyors who evaluate pressure ulcer care in LTC facilities.[2] The term *pressure ulcer* is preferable to *bed sore* or *decubitus ulcer* because it describes the cause. The initial appearance is a pressure area (Figure 18). Many LTC residents have problems with impaired circulation, impaired sensation, poor nutrition, and edema from multiple causes, which are contributing factors. From a small pressure area in the foot, a cascade of problems

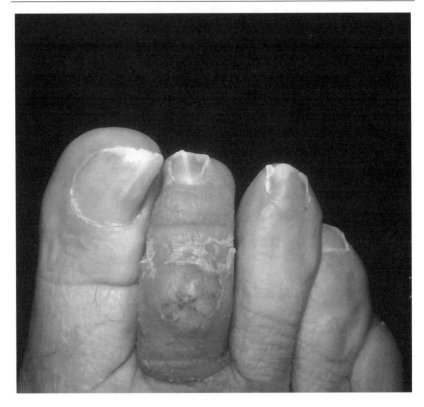

Figure 18.   Earliest sign of an ulcer (also hammertoe, heloma, and fusiform deformity [arthritis]).

can develop and result in an ulcer (Figures 19–21). Unfortunately in some cases, amputation can follow. The national prevalence for pressure ulcers in LTC is approximately 9.9%.[2] Data from the National Pressure Ulcer Advisory Panel have noted the incidence of pressure ulcers in LTC facilities to range from 2.2% to 23.9%. The Centers for Medicare and Medicaid Services (CMS) established the reduction of pressure ulcers as one of its goals for the Government Performance Results Acts (GPRA) in LTC facilities. CMS has mandated that each state Quality Improvement Organization deal with the problem of pressure ulcers in these facilities; furthermore, CMS believes that this complication can be decreased.[2, 3]

Many LTC residents have problems communicating because of varying degrees of dementia and hearing and visual problems. There-

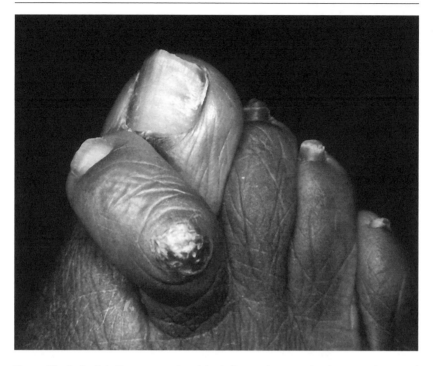

Figure 19. Early diabetic pressure ulcer (also hallaux valgus, overlapping second toe, and heloma).

fore, LTC professionals cannot rely on the residents to report symptoms of pressure areas. Furthermore, because of impaired sensation in the feet primarily as a result of diabetic neuropathy, symptoms may not be present. All of the professional providers in LTC facilities must be in constant communication with patients as well as families before and after problems develop so that they can be warned about the possibility of these complications. With increasing degrees of immobility, there are more chances for pressure problems.

Because litigation unfortunately is not unusual in the United States, detailed documentation in the medical record is mandatory. The record should include measures that were taken before and after a pressure area was noted and methods that were used to prevent progression.

Pressure ulcers indeed are a big deal. When a pressure ulcer develops within 3 months of admission to a LTC facility, there is a 92%

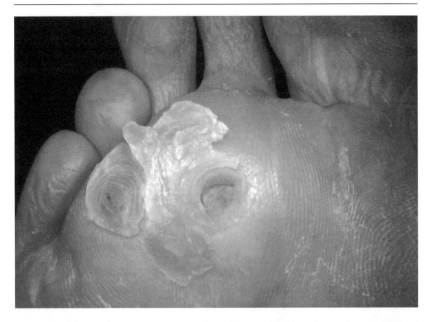

Figure 20. Ulcer (pressure) at an advancing stage (also marginal hyperkeratosis and peripheral arterial disease).

mortality rate as compared with a mortality rate of 4% in residents who did not develop a pressure ulcer.[2] Significantly increased mortality of residents with pressure ulcers in LTC facilities occurs after 6 months: 77.3% with ulcers versus 18.7%.[4] Healing of pressure ulcers conversely improves mortality figures: 11% versus 64%.[5] These figures clearly indicate that pressure ulcers are a marker for risk of frailty in older adults; therefore, prevention and management should focus on these systemic problems, some of which are correctable.

The vast majority of diabetic foot complications that result in amputation begin with the formation of skin ulcers. More than 70% of foot amputations are due to complicated foot ulcers. Early detection and appropriate treatment of these ulcers may prevent up to 85% of these amputations.[6, 7, 8]

Pressure ulcers in individuals with diabetes are the most common problem that leads to lower extremity amputation.[9] These are problems of older adults: More than 50% of people with pressure ulcers are 70 years and older. Furthermore, as many as 20% to 33% of individuals who are admitted to nursing facilities have a significant

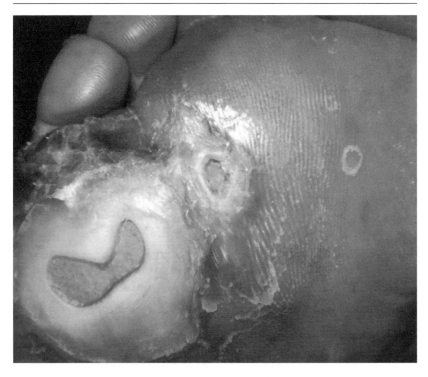

Figure 21. Advanced-stage pressure ulcers (also marginal keratosis and early necrosis).

pressure ulcer.[10] This information indicates how pervasive these problems are in older adults.

CAUSE OF PRESSURE ULCERS

Pressure and shear force are the primary causative factors. Shearing force is generated by any circumstance whereby the body and parts of the body are slid over surfaces. For example, when the head of the bed is elevated and the body slides down, shear force is created. Friction is another factor, such as when a person is pulled across bed sheets or when feet or other parts of the body slide over rough surfaces. Moisture, urine, feces, and sweating will increase the possibility of pressure problems as a result of maceration of the tissues. All individuals who are at risk should have a systematic skin inspection at least once a day, with particular attention paid to the bony prominences. Results of skin inspection should be documented.

PREVENTION

Identifying high-risk residents is key to preventing pressure ulcers. Residents who are confined to a bed are at high risk. Those with poor nutrition, edema, impaired circulation, and diabetes also are at high risk. Residents who largely are confined to wheelchairs are next at risk for development of pressure problems. Quality nursing care is the first line of defense in preventing pressure ulcers.

All types of particulate matter, such as food, paper, and so forth, should be removed from the bed. Sheets should be loose so that movement is not restricted. Residents should be lifted, not dragged across surfaces; use lifting devices such as a trapeze or bed linen to move rather than drag individuals who cannot assist during transfers or position changes. The skin should be patted dry, not rubbed. The head of the bed should not be raised to more than 30 degrees to avoid shear force that is generated by the body's sliding toward the foot of the bed. The upright position should be maintained when a resident is in a wheelchair. Sheepskin pads can be used to avoid shear resistance.

Rotation and change of position in residents who are confined to a bed should occur every 2 hours. Careful inspection of problem areas in the feet should be conducted at least twice daily. Also, if the resident has antithrombotic stockings, then these should be removed for inspection of the skin areas in the feet. Use pillows as bridging to prevent pressure problems. Careful inspection of the calves is necessary when pillows are placed in this location to avoid pressure areas in the feet.

Discussion of special devices to relieve pressure and shear are beyond the scope of this chapter. Usually, the management staff of LTC facilities is responsible for the investigation, evaluation, and purchase of these devices.

There are several types of mattresses. Active mattresses include low air loss (SAR Low Air Loss Mattress System) or alternating air system. Passive mattresses, including Sof-care or "egg-crate" styles, are reserved for residents who can reposition themselves independently or on command. Less effective for pressure reduction and available at a lower price are foam mattresses.

Residents sitting in wheelchairs present a different problem. Particular attention must be paid to residents who lack sensation and cannot shift weight independently. In these cases, the sacral and buttock areas are the major risk sites. Because of its thin layer of subcutaneous tissue between skin and bone, the heel is the most common site for pressure ulcer development after the sacrum, accounting for 30% of pressure ulcers.[11]

MANAGEMENT

In LTC facilities, pain is the fourth vital sign. Aside from peripheral neuropathy, pain from pressure areas and ulcers is significant. Residents with cognitive problems do indeed experience pain. LTC personnel must inquire about pain just as they would measure the other vital signs. Once a pressure area develops, general measures to promote wound healing should be instituted with physician involvement. Increasing protein intake can promote wound healing. In this situation, consultation with a dietitian is mandatory. Correction of edema, anemia, and hypoxemia will promote wound healing with appropriate physician participation.

Residents with diabetes pose a special problem. The risk for amputation of a lower extremity increases 25% with each 1% rise in glycosylated hemoglobin above normal. The goal of wound debridement is to remove dead tissue, which, if not removed, promotes infection and delays granulation and therefore delays healing. Wound debridement can be mechanical, chemical, or surgical.

Mechanical debridement is accomplished with wet-to-dry dressing, by using fine-mesh gauze soaked in normal saline solution and loosely packed in the wound, with removal every 3 to 4 hours. For prevention of pain and reduction of the damage to granulation and epithelial tissue, saline solution may be applied to loosen the contact layer of gauze if it adheres to the wound. A number of agents have been developed to provide chemical debridement (collagenase, sutilains, fibrinolysin, streptokinase, and trypsin-papain). A silver sulfadiazine (silverdine) frequently is used to soften an eschar and reduce bacterial count. The most promising agents are an adhesive hydrocolloid occlusive dressing (DuoDERM) and a polyurethane film dressing.

In all stages of management of pressure ulcers, physicians' involvement is necessary concerning the use of systemic antibiotics, local antibiotics, and other local measures. However, the hour-to-hour, day-to-day care is the responsibility of the nursing staff of LTC facilities.

For help in determining which residents are most likely to develop pressure ulcers, the mnemonic device *DECUBITUS* is suggested:

- **D** for **d**elirium, **d**ementia, and **d**ependence: Only an individual with a clear mind can act purposefully to relieve a noxious stimulus. Therefore, residents with altered mental status, such as coma or severe dementia, are at risk for skin breakdown. Residents who are at risk for pressure ulcers are partially or completely dependent on others. Residents who require one or two people to assist them in getting into bed are at high risk for ulceration.

- **E** for **e**lderly. Seventy percent of pressure ulcers occur in older adults. Frailty, dependence, incontinence, chronic illnesses, and degenerative neurological diseases increase with age. Associated with aging are diminished pain perception and blunting of the inflammatory response. Histologic changes in skin include flattening of the dermal–epidermal junction and reduced elastin content, both of which increase susceptibility to shear and minor laceration. Ulcer closure is delayed because of reduced rates of both reepithelialization and contraction.

- **C** for **c**ontractures: When severe, contractures prevent routine turning and positioning on most mattress types. Contractures increase point pressure and therefore contribute to delayed healing and increased incidence of pressure ulcers.

- **U** for **u**rinary incontinence: Wet skin is macerated easily. When the urine is infected, the skin and any ulcers will be contaminated.

- **B** for **b**owel incontinence: Soiling may lead to bacterial colonization or local infection. The wet skin that is associated with diarrhea also contributes to ulcer formation.

- **I** for **i**mmobility: Long-term bed rest leads to a decrease in lean muscle mass of 5% per week and contributes to osteoporosis and contractures through collagen remodeling within tendons and joint capsules. Immobility feeds a vicious cycle of wasting, contractures, pressure "hot spots," and worsening ulceration.

- **T** for **t**ension O_2 low (a decrease in oxygen in the tissue, retarding wound healing): Ischemia is related to ulcer formation. Anemia should be corrected (e.g., by iron supplementation). Edema impairs gas and nutrient exchange between healing tissue and the blood supply.

- **U** for **u**ndernourishment: Inadequate caloric or protein intake may result in malnutrition and impaired ulcer healing.

- **S** for **s**pasticity, **s**ensory loss, and **s**pinal cord injury: By several mechanisms, neurological injury predisposes to pressure ulcer formation:

Spasticity (increased muscle tone) predisposes to contracture formation and poor mobility.

Lack of protective sensation, which leads to pressure ulcer formation, may be dermatomal with spinal cord injury or hemisensory with stroke.

Spinal cord injury, especially above T6, is related to sympathetic nervous system dysfunction and impaired skin perfusion at the site of pressure[11]

REFERENCES

[1]Lyder, C.H. (2006). Implication of pressure ulcers and its relation to federal tag 314. *Annals of Long Term Care: Clinical Care and Aging, 14,* 19–24.

[2]Center for Medicare and Medicaid Services. (2004, December). *Action plan for further improvement of nursing home quality.* Retrieved June 5, 2006, from http://www.cms.hhs.gov/CertificationandComplianc/downloads/2005NHActionPlan.pdf

[3]Cuddington, J., Ayello, E.A., Sussman, C., & Branaski, S. (Eds.). (2001). *Pressure ulcers in America: Prevalence, incidence, and implications for the future.* Reston, VA: National Pressure Ulcer Advisory Panel.

[4]Thomas, A. (1992). Managing pressure ulcer risk in long-term care. *Nursing Homes, 51,* 66.

[5]Bergstrom, N., & Braden, B. (1992). A prospective study of pressure sore risk among institutionalized elderly. *Journal of the American Geriatrics Society, 40,* 747–758.

[6]Brandeis, G.H., Morris, S.N., Nash, D.J., & Lipsitz, L.H. (1990). The epidemiology and natural history of pressure ulcers in elderly nursing home residents. *Journal of the American Medical Association, 264,* 2905–2909

[7]Reed, J.W. (1981). Pressure ulcers in the elderly: prevention and treatment utilizing the team approach. *Maryland State Medical Journal, 130,* 45–50.

[8] Black, J. (2004). Preventing heel pressure ulcers. *Nursing, 34,* 17.

[9]Thomas, D.R. (2003). Management of chronic wounds. In C.K. Cassel, R.M. Leipzig, H.G. Cohen, E.B. Larson, & D.E. Meier (Eds.), *Geriatric medicine* (4th ed., pp. 519–527). New York: Springer-Verlag.

[10]United States National Diabetes Advisory Board. (1987). *The national long-range plan to combat diabetes* (NIH Publication No. 88-1587). Bethesda, MD: U.S. Department of Health and Human Services, Public Health Service, National Institutes of Health.

[11]Goldman, R. (2004). Pressure ulcers. In M.A. Forciea, R. Lavizzo-Mourey, E.P. Schwab, & D.B Raziano (Eds.), *Geriatric secrets* (3rd ed., pp. 276–277). Philadelphia: Hanely and Belfus.

CHAPTER SEVEN

Foot Health and Falls in the Long-Term Care Resident

Roberta A. Newton

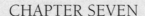

T he ability to maintain mobility—regardless of physical, cognitive, and residency status—is extremely important for older adults and their caregivers. This chapter reviews literature that pertains to the foot and falls and provides select assessments and preventive strategies for front-line practitioners to reduce falls in the long-term care (LTC) environment.

Mood, sudden and ongoing illnesses and conditions, and cognitive status affect posture of the body, the alignment of the body to the foot, and the relationship of the foot to the floor during standing, walking, and other locomotor activities. The foot needs to accommodate static and dynamic body postures and the interaction of the individual with the environment during daily activities.

The foot and the ankle need to be flexible to absorb the shock of impact as the heel hits the ground as well as to provide stability as the person shifts weight from heel contact to toe-off during walking or performing other activities. In addition, the foot and the ankle need to be flexible to adapt to uneven surfaces during walking. During performance of activities of daily living that require standing, the foot and the ankle need to be able to accept weight when the person shifts side to side, leans forward and backward, reaches up or down, or rotates the body. The foot and the ankle need to be flexible to accommodate partial weight bearing of the foot, which occurs during standing or balancing on the balls of the feet or walking up the stairs when the entire foot is not placed on the step.

FALLS AND FALL-RELATED INJURIES IN THE LONG-TERM CARE ENVIRONMENT

The figures related to falls and fall-related injuries among older adults who live in the community and LTC environments demonstrate that falls represent a major public health care concern. Incidence rates for community-dwelling older adults generally show that 30% to 40% fall annually. The number of falls may be higher than actually reported as a result of forgetting to report a fall, reporting a slip or trip instead of the fall, and fear of the loss of independence. A higher incidence rate is noted for hospitalized and institutionalized older adults (Table 1).

Unintentional falls in the LTC environment have been defined as "unintentionally coming to rest on the ground, floor, or other lower level but not as a result of an overwhelming external force (e.g., resident pushes another resident). An episode where a resident lost his/her balance and would have fallen, if not for staff intervention, is considered a fall. A fall without injury is still a fall. Unless there is evidence suggesting otherwise, when a resident is found on the floor, a fall is considered to have occurred" (L.B. Goldman, personal communication, December 13, 2005).

When comparing LTC resident with community-dwelling older adult fall rates, the higher rate for residents may be due to better documenting of falls in the hospital or nursing facility and residents who 1) are older, 2) have more ongoing health conditions, 3) have more limitations in routine activities of daily living, 4) may have more cog-

Table 1. Statistics associated with falls among older adults who are hospitalized or who reside in a nursing facility

Hospital setting: Annual incidence rate is approximately 1.4 falls per bed per year (range 0.5–2.7 falls).
The departments of neuroscience, rehabilitation, and psychiatry have the highest rates, ranging from 8.9 to 17.1 falls per 1000 patient-days.[1]
LTC facility: Annual incidence rate is approximately 1.6 falls per bed annually (range 0.2–3.6 falls).[2]
Nursing facility residents: Approximately 43% of the residents fall each year (range 16%–75%). Residents often experience multiple falls, averaging 2.6 falls per person per year.[3]
Approximately 10% to 20% of all falls in a nursing facility cause serious injuries, and approximately 2% to 6% result in fractures.
Approximately 35% of fall-related injuries occur among the nonambulatory residents.[4]

[1]Nyberg, Gustafson, Janson, Sandman, and Eriksson (1997).
[2]Rubenstein and Powers (1999).
[3]Rubenstein, Josephson, and Robbins (1994).
[4]Thapa, Brockman, Gideon, Fought, and Ray (1996).

nitive impairment, and 5) tend to be more frail than community-dwelling older adults.[5, 6, 7] As noted in Table 1, the ranges of reported falls vary and may be due to several factors: case mix, ambulatory level of the older adult, method(s) for reporting a fall, and the method(s) used to calculate fall rates. Most striking is that approximately 20% of all fall-related deaths among older adults occur among the 5% who live in nursing facilities.[8] This figure translates into approximately 1800 fatal falls occurring among residents of U.S. nursing facilities each year. In 1997, 1.5 million people 65 years and older lived in nursing facilities[9]; this figure is expected to rise to 3 million by 2030.[10] A proportional increase in fall incidence, fall-related injuries, and fall-related deaths also is expected. Two of the major risk factors associated with falls are impairments in balance and gait. The foot is a major contributor to maintenance of good balance and gait.

IMPORTANCE OF THE FOOT
IN BALANCE AND WALKING

Balance is the ability of a person to maintain his or her center of mass (COM) over the base of support when a person is standing still or moving about in the environment.[11] The base of support (BOS) is defined by the boundaries of the feet. When a person stands with feet close together, the BOS is narrower than the person's typical stance. When a person stands with feet wider apart, the BOS is wider than the person's typical stance. Having a narrower BOS by placing the feet closer together or standing with more weight on one leg tends to be a more unstable position. If a person habitually stands with more weight on one leg, then this is the preferred stance position. The BOS can be increased if the person uses a cane or a walker. The use of an assistive device such as a cane or a walker increases balance stability.[12]

Sensory systems—such as the vision system, the vestibular system, and the somatosensory system of the feet—provide information to the brain about the external environment. The somatosensory system of the feet consists of cutaneous receptors and proprioceptors that monitor temperature, pressure, pain, and location of the joints of the ankle and the feet. These sensory systems provide information about lighting, location of objects, and the condition of the support surface (e.g., floor). As older adults stand or move about in the environment (monitored by the vestibular system), it is important for them to have accurate knowledge about the conditions of the support surface— that is, whether the surface is hard or compliant, slippery or dry, level or uneven. Besides looking at the support surface, valuable information about the support surface is picked up from sensory receptors in the feet and transmitted to the brain. On the basis of all sensory input and past experiences, the brain selects appropriate balance or movement strategies so that the individual can navigate safely in the environment without falling.

Medical conditions such as peripheral vascular disease and diabetes can affect the somatosensory system of the lower extremity and the foot. As a result, the older adult has a decreased capability to detect the conditions of the support surface, thereby increasing the risk for falls. Only recently has diabetes been recognized as an important risk factor for falls. Mauer et al.[13] followed 139 nursing facility residents for 299 days and noted that 78% of the residents with diabetes fell compared with 30% of those without diabetes.

Menz and Lord[14] examined the effect of foot problems on the ability of community-dwelling older adults to perform various functional tasks. Eighty-seven percent of the older adults had at least one foot problem, such as digit deformity, foot pain, hallux valgus, and plantar hyperkeratosis. The researchers noted that those with foot pain performed worse in challenging balance tasks and functional tasks such as alternate step-up test, stair ascent and descent, and the timed 6-meter walk test. Older adults with painful feet or decreased sensation in the feet alter their posture and walking pattern in an attempt to relieve the foot pain and to remain ambulatory. Such alteration of gait, posture, and stability leads to balance instability and fall risk. Foot pain can be reduced by intervention, thereby maintaining or increasing mobility of the older adult.

When alterations of the normal coordination of the ankle and the foot occur, the associated biomechanical changes have a profound affect on other structures. For example, foot and ankle malalignment over time can result in symptoms of knee and hip stress. The result is a cycle of altered postural alignment, increased stress and pain, and decreased activity in an attempt to relieve pain. Such a cycle reduces mobility of the older adult and places the person at greater risk for falls and other health conditions as a result of immobility. This cycle results in greater impairment and function decline in older adult residents in LTC environments.

FOOTWEAR AND FALL RISK IN OLDER ADULTS

Many intrinsic (self) and extrinsic (environmental) risk factors have been identified for falls.[15, 16] Two risk factors that tend to be overlooked are foot health and footwear. Footwear may contribute to falls through several mechanisms; for example, the sole and the tread may have either increased or decreased friction, causing a risk for slipping or tripping.[17, 19] Height and width of shoe and fit of the shoe[20] also may cause instability in balance and gait. For example high heels may cause lateral instability and decrease stride length.[21] The thickness of the toe box can decrease the amount of toe clearance when the foot is brought forward during the swing phase of gait, thereby causing the shoe to "catch" on the support surface and causing the person to trip or stumble. The weight of the shoe also may be a factor for fall risk in frail older adults or older adults of short stature (R.A.N., unpublished observations, 2003).

The thickness of the shoe can affect the ability of the sensory receptors in the feet to sense the support surface. This is of particular

Table 2.   Fall risk and footwear

	Odds ratio	95% confidence interval
Stocking feet/barefoot[a]	10.2	3–35
Stocking feet	5.5	1.5–20.7
High-heel shoes	2.8	.8–6.8
Slippers	1.3	.7–2.4
Flats	2.0	.7–4.6
Sandals and loafers	1.4	.6–3.2 (sandals) .7–2.5 (loafers)
Tie shoes (oxfords)	1.2	.8–1.9
Canvas shoes	.9	.4–1.9
Athletic shoes	1.0	reference

From Koepsell, T.D., Wolf, M.E., Buchner, D.M., Kukull, W.A., LaCroiz, A.Z., Tencer, A.F., et al. (2004). Footwear style and risk of falls in older adults. *Journal of the American Geriatrics Society, 52,* 1498; adapted by permission.

[a]Odds ratio calculated when footwear was grouped into three categories: shoeless, athletic/canvas shoes, and other shoewear.

consideration because older adults have decreased responsiveness of the somatosensory receptors as a result of aging or thickness of the callus on the soles of the feet.

Koepsell and colleagues monitored falls in 1,371 older adults for 2 years.[18] Those who fell were asked about footwear at the time of the fall. In this study, most older adults wore athletic shoes. The researchers noted that wearing athletic or canvas shoes resulted in a lower risk factor. Barefoot or stocking feet compared with athletic or canvas shoes were associated with a 10.2-fold increase in the risk for a fall. When compared with athletic or canvas shoes, other footwear demonstrated a 1.3-fold increase in a risk for a fall. High heels and slippers also would be considered risk factors for falls (see Table 2).

On the basis of these findings, however, practitioners should not recommend immediate discontinuation of the wearing of high heels. Older adults who have worn high heels throughout their lives have shortened gastrocnemius/soleus (calf) muscles. This position shifts the COM forward in the BOS. Immediately dispensing with the high heels would create pain in the calf muscles as a result of stretching and create a fall risk because of the perception of falling backward (the COM has shifted toward the back of the BOS). Two interventions are recommended: 1) gradually reducing heel height over time and 2) having the person wear a larger size heel to increase heel stability with the ultimate goal of increasing stability and reducing fall risk.

ASSESSMENT OF THE FOOT IN RELATION TO FALLS FOR FRONT-LINE PRACTITIONERS

Foot assessment should be included as part of each practitioner's assessment of the older adult, particularly when the older adult is immobile, has recurrent falls, or has a medical condition that affects the vascular status and biomechanical alignment of the ankle and the foot (e.g., orthopedic and neurological conditions).

The foot assessment should address risk factors for falls. Areas assessed include foot and ankle range of motion and sensation, lower limb strength, balance, and mobility. General observation of the foot and the shoe is recommended.

Foot and ankle range of motion and strength are important elements for balance, stability, and mobility. Older adults, particularly those who are sedentary, have a decrease in both plantarflexor and dorsiflexor strength. A decrease in muscle strength coupled with a decrease in foot and ankle range of motion limits the ability of the foot and ankle complex to adapt to changing walking surfaces. Separate testing of range of motion and muscle strength can be conducted; however, a general indication of range of motion and muscle strength can be observed during physical performance testing.

Reliable and valid measurement batteries are used to assess physical performance in residents in the LTC environment. These measures include but are not limited to the Physical Disability Index (PDI; see Table 3),[22] the Physical Performance and Mobility Examination,[23] the Epidemiologic Study of the Elderly (EPSE) battery,[24] the Tinetti-Performance Oriented Examination,[25] and the Berg Balance Test.[26]

Additional measures to document balance and gait include clinical measures[27] such as the Multi-Directional Reach Test[28] and the Timed Up and Go test.[29] An instrumented system such as the GaitRite (http://www.gaitrite.com) documents various parameters of gait, including the gait stability ratio,[30] speed, cadence, and step width and length; the NeuroCom Smart Balance (http://www.onbalance.com/)

Table 3.   Items of the Physical Disability Index (PDI)

1.   Range of motion in the upper and lower extremities
2.   Strength of the upper and lower extremities
3.   Balance tests: sit unassisted, stand up from a chair, stand with feet in various positions (apart, together, semitandem, tandem)
4.   Mobility including bed mobility, chair transfer, turn 180 degrees, walk for 50 feet

Source: Gerety M.B., Mulrow C.D., Tuley M.R., Hazuda, H.P., Lichtenstein, M.J., Bohannon, R., et al. (1993).

system is used to document balance, including location of the COM in relation to the BOS, the amount of sway in standing, and the ability to maintain balance during tasks such as head turning.

Observational analysis of the foot and the ankle during walking also is useful to determine whether the individual places an appropriate amount of weight on the foot and uses a typical heel-to-toe pattern of floor contact during walking. Family members and caregivers can provide empirical evidence about balance stability and walking.

Sensation

A general foot assessment for front-line health care workers includes, for example, the following:

- Observation of the skin for dryness and calluses, hair growth and color, and overgrown toenails
- Detection and documentation of the presence of redness or ulcers
- Determination of location of pain by asking the person to point to where the foot "hurts" or indicate location of pain on a foot diagram
- Cutaneous sensation using Semmes-Weinstein monofilaments (the monofilaments measure the perception from light touch to loss of protective sensation)
- Bony alignment of the foot for lesser toe deformities such as hammertoes and overlapping toes
- Pulses

A general inspection of the shoe includes, for example, the following:

- Examination of the pattern of wear on the sole, heel, and lateral border of the shoe

- Examination of the inside of the shoe for wear patterns, particularly as it relates to reddened areas or ulcers on the foot. A rule of thumb for proper shoe fit is that with the older adult standing, the practitioner's thumb should fit between the longest toe and the end of the older adult's shoe and a slight give should be felt before the metatarsal heads are felt when the practitioner squeezes the shoe at the level of the metatarsal heads. A potential for rubbing and developing ulcers may occur if the metatarsal heads are in contact with the lateral borders of the toe box.

- Observation of whether socks/stockings are a good fit and are clean

- Checking for foot hygiene and use of appropriate supplements (e.g., lotion)

PREVENTIVE STRATEGIES FOR THE FOOT IN RELATION TO FALLS FOR FRONT-LINE PRACTITIONERS

Many preventive strategies to reduce fall risk exist. This section provides examples of some strategies to maintain good foot health to reduce the chances for falls.

A Daily Foot Check that Can Be Performed by the Older Adult or Caregiver

Depending on the physical and cognitive status of the older adult and the caregiver, each person can be empowered to assist with a daily foot check. This check does not obviate the responsibility of the practitioner to perform the daily check. Figure 22 is an example of a foot check for the older adult or the caregiver. The foot check and general

---

Check Those Toes: Daily Foot Checklist

1. Do you have:
   - Clean feet to put into a pair of clean socks?
   - Good fitting shoes to wear today?
2. Do you have:
   - Loss of feeling or feet that burn or tingle?
   - Redness, blisters, dryness, or cracks between your toes?
   - An infection or an open area on your foot?
   - Corns or calluses that cause you pain or discomfort?
   - Cramps or hurting in your legs or feet when you walk, sit, or are in bed at night?
   - Have toenails that are ingrown, are thickened, or have changed shape?
3. Did you check the bottom of your feet?
   - Use a mirror to help you see the bottom of your feet, or get someone to look at the bottom of your feet.

   If you find any unusual change in your feet, report it to your primary care doctor and your foot doctor (podiatrist) right away.

   Good feet, good health!

Figure 22. Sample of a foot checklist for an older adult or a caregiver. (From Newton, R.A. [2004].*The Fall Prevention Program manual.* Retrieved June 5, 2006, from http://www.temple .edu/older_adult/fppmanual.html; adapted by permission.)

care tips can hang on the refrigerator door or other visible area (bathroom door knob) as a reminder to "check those toes."

Medication Review

Medication management is important to maintain the health of the individual. Polypharmacy (taking multiple medications) may increase the risk for a stumble or a fall. The interaction of medications may cause, for example, dizziness, drowsiness, or hypotension. Review of all medications is an important strategy.

Documentation of the Fall

In addition to the standard documentation of falls, the assessment of footwear should be included. Some LTC facilities recommend a specific type of footwear for all residents.

Activity Program

An activity program can be established to maintain balance, mobility, flexibility, and range of motion. Activities can include, for example, walking, dancing, and chair exercises that are at the appropriate level for the resident.

Environmental Modification

Environmental modification includes, for example, the following:

- A support surface that is nonskid, nonglare, and obstacle-free so that the resident does not slip, trip, or fall

- A support surface that is level and free of uneven sections

- Arrangement of furniture so that the resident's feet do not catch in the legs of the furniture or under the furniture.

Education of the Staff

Educational topics for the staff include good foot health, care of the feet, medical conditions that decrease sensation of the feet, body alignment in relation to the feet, footwear and care, safe transfers, and ambulation to keep older adults mobile.[31, 32]

CONCLUSION

Foot health is an important part of maintaining mobility in older adults. Good foot health and appropriate footwear are factors that can reduce the risk for falls in older adults.

REFERENCES

[1]Nyberg, L., Gustafson, Y., Janson, A., Sandman, P.O., & Eriksson, S. (1997). Incidence of falls in three different types of geriatric care. *Scandinavian Journal of Social Medicine, 25,* 8–13.

[2]Rubenstein, L.Z., & Powers, C. (1999). *Falls and mobility problems: Potential quality indicators and literature review (the ACOVE Project)* (pp. 1–40). Santa Monica, CA: RAND Corporation.

[3]Rubenstein, L.Z., Josephson, K.R., & Robbins, A.S. (1994). Falls in the nursing home. *Annals of Internal Medicine, 121,* 442–451.

[4]Thapa, P.B., Brockman, K.G., Gideon, P., Fought, R.L., & Ray, W.A. (1996). Injurious falls in nonambulatory nursing home residents: A comparative study of circumstances, incidence and risk factors. *Journal of the American Geriatrics Society, 44,* 273–278.

[5]Janitti, P.O., Pyykko, I., & Laippala, P. (1995). Prognosis of falls among elderly nursing home residents. *Aging: Clinical and Experimental Research, 7,* 23–27.

[6]Tinetti, M.E., Liu, W.L., & Ginter, S.F. (1992). Mechanical restraint use and fall-related injuries among residents of skilled nursing facilities. *Annals of Internal Medicine, 116,,* 369–374.

[7]Basante, J., Bentz, E., Eeck-Hackley, J., Kenion, B., Young, D., & Holm, M.B. (2001). Fall risk among older adults in long-term care facilities: A focused literature review. *Physical & Occupational Therapy in Geriatrics, 19,* 63–85.

[8]Rubenstein, L.Z. (1997). Preventing falls in the nursing home. *Journal of the American Medical Association, 278,* 595–596.

[9]Kramarow, E., Lentzner, H., Rooks, R., Weeks, J., & Saydah, S. (1999). *Health and aging chartbook: Health, United States, 1999.* Hyattsville, MD: National Center for Health Statistics.

[10]Sahyoun, N.R., Pratt, L.A., Lentzner, H., Dey, A., & Robinson, K.N. (2001). *The changing profile of nursing home residents: 1985–1997: Aging trends; No. 4.* Hyattsville, MD: National Center for Health Statistics.

[11]Newton, R.A. (2003). Balance and falls among older people. *Generations, 27,* 27–31.

[12]Bateni, H., & Maki, B. (2005). Assistive devices for balance and mobility: Benefits, demands, and adverse consequences. *Archives of Physical Medicine and Rehabilitation, 86,* 134–45.

[13]Mauer, M.S., Burcham, J., & Cheng, H. (2005). Diabetes mellitus is associated with an increased risk of falls in elderly residents of a long-term care facility. *Journal of Gerontology, 60A,* 1157–1162.

[14]Menz, H.B., & Lord, S.R. (2001) Foot pain impairs balance and functional ability in community-dwelling older people. *Journal of the American Podiatric Medical Association, 91,* 222–229.

[15]Rubenstein, L.Z., & Josephson, K.R. (2002). The epidemiology of falls and syncope. *Clinics in Geriatric Medicine, 18,* 141–158.

[16]Lipsitz, R.M., Cumming, R.G., & Tinetti, M.E. (1999). Drugs and falls in older people. A systematic review and meta-analysis: I. Psychotropic drugs. II. Cardiac and analgesic drugs. *Journal of the American Geriatrics Society, 47,* 30–50.

[17]Frey, C., & Kubasak, M. (1998). Faulty footwear contributes to why senior citizens fall. *Biomechanics, 5,* 45–48.

[18]Koepsell, T.D., Wolf, M.E., Buchner, D.M., Kukull, W.A., LaCroiz, A.Z., Tencer, A.F., et al. (2004). Footwear style and risk of falls in older adults. *Journal of the American Geriatrics Society, 52,* 1495–1501.

[19]Tencer, A.F., Koepsell, T.D., Wolf, M.E., Frankenfeld, C.L., Buchner, D.M., Kukull, W.A., et al. (2004). Biomechanical properties of shoes and risk of falls in older adults. *Journal of the American Geriatrics Society, 52,* 1840–1846.

[20]Frey, C. (2000). Foot health and shoewear for women. *Clinical Orthopaedics and Related Research, 372,* 32–44.

[21]Adrian, M.J., & Karpovich, P.V. (1966). Foot instability during walking in shoes with high heels. *Research Quarterly, 37,* 168–175.

[22]Bohannon, R., et al. (1993). Development and validation of a physical performance instrument for the functionally impaired elderly: The Physical Disability Index (PDI). *Journal of Gerontology, 48,* M33–M38.

[23]Winograd, C.H., Lemsky, C.M., Nevitt, M.C., Nordstrom, T.M., Stewart, A.L., Miller, C.J., et al. (1994). Development of a physical performance and mobility examination. *Journal of the American Geriatrics Society, 42,* 743–749.

[24]Guralnik, J.M., Simonsick, E.M., Ferrucci, L., Glynn, R.J., Berkman, L.F., Blazer, D.G., et al. (1994). A short physical performance battery assessing lower extremity function: Association with self-reported disability and prediction of mortality and nursing home admission. *Journal of Gerontology, 49,* M85–M94.

[25]Tinetti, M.E. (1986). Performance-oriented assessment of mobility problems in elderly adults. *Journal of the American Geriatrics Society, 34* 119–126.

[26]Berg, K.O., Wood-Dauphine, S.L., Williams, J.T., & Maki, B.E. (1992). Measuring balance in the elderly: validation of an instrument. *Canadian Journal of Public Health, 83,* S7–S11.

[27]Harada, N., Chiu, V., Damron-Rodriguez, J., Fowler, E., Siu, A., & Reuben, D.B. (1995). Screening for balance and mobility impairment in elderly individuals living in residential care facilities. *Physical Therapy, 75*(6), 462–469

[28]Newton, R.A. (2001). Validity of the multi-directional reach test: A practical measure for limits of stability in older adults. *Journal of Gerontology, 56*(3), M248–M252.

[29]Podsiadlo, D., & Richardson, S. (1991). The timed "Up and Go" test: A test of basic functional mobility for frail elderly persons. *Journal of the American Geriatrics Society, 39,* 142–148.

[30]Cromwell, R.L., & Newton, R.A. (2004). Relationship between balance and gait stability in healthy older adults. *Journal of Aging and Physical Activity, 12,* 90–100.

[31]Newton, R.A. (2004). *HEROS© Reducing Falls and Serious Injuries: Training program manual.* Retrieved June 5, 2006, from http://www.temple.edu/ older_adult

[32]American Medical Directors Association. (2003). *Clinical practice guideline: Falls and fall risk.* Retrieved June 5, 2006, from http://www.amda .com/info/cpg/falls.htm

CHAPTER EIGHT

Basic Considerations for Geriatric Footwear

The interest in footwear for older adults surfaced as a significant issue with the adoption of the Medicare Therapeutic Shoe Bill of 1993. The requirements provide allowed reimbursement for Medicare-eligible patients who have diabetes and have one or more of the conditions listed in the Appendix. In addition, the patient must be under a comprehensive plan of care by a medical physician (M.D., D.O.) for diabetes. The patient also must need special shoes (depth or custom molded) because of diabetes.

For the purposes of Medicare and as a general requirement, a custom-molded shoe is constructed over a cast, or model, of the patient's foot. It has to be made of leather or another suitable material of equal quality and must have some form of closure, such as laces or Velcro. The custom shoe also must have inserts that can be removed, altered, or replaced, according to the individual's conditions and needs. A depth shoe has an insole, or a filler, that extends from heel to toe and provides at least $\frac{3}{16}''$ of additional depth when removed. An extra-depth shoe provides $\frac{1}{4}''$ of additional depth, and a super-depth shoe provides $\frac{1}{2}''$ of additional depth for total-contact orthoses, or inserts.

It is clear to clinicians that for many older adults who are equally at risk for other conditions, such as arterial insufficiency, rheumatoid and degenerative arthritis, gout, and other conditions of the neurological and musculoskeletal systems, footwear holds a direct relationship to foot problems. It must be remembered that shoes alone do not cause foot problems, but shoe-to-foot incompatibilities do help to precipitate pressure areas, pain, and limitation of ambulation and require the same careful selection for the individual without diabetes as for the individual with diabetes.

The human foot is an organ that is both static and mobile. It provides support for the body at rest and during propulsion and ambulation. For the older adult, the ability to remain mobile and functional often is the key to quality of life, performing activities and instrumental activities of daily living, and continuing to live in the community.

In addition to its static and propulsive activity, the human foot is subjected to forces and activities by the changes in society, such as hard, flat walking surfaces and the forces of gravity, which are related to the weight and the activity level of the individual as well as the changes in muscular activity related to function, motion, and disability. With the older adult, gait dysfunction and osseous remodeling (changes in bone structure) are related to the resilience of the foot itself and the foot's ability to respond and adapt to stress. Footwear for the older adult must function as an integral part of activity and become an extension of the individual.

The foot, from a morphologic standpoint, basically is a modified rectangle. When disease and/or deformity is present, the changes that occur may alter the sides of the rectangle, but the basic figure is retained. It also should be noted that the foot is three-dimensional and that this must be a consideration in all footwear, modifications, and related orthotics. Issues that must be considered include loading; stance; propulsion; and gait and speed and their interaction to the shoe, which in a sense, is an article of protective clothing.

The shoes that are provided to older adults must be appropriate for the activity that is being undertaken and must assist not only in protection but also in helping to reduce shear and shock and to assist in the transfer of force from one part of the foot to another during the gait cycle and during stance. In addition, shoes should not produce pain and discomfort but can be modified or combined with orthotics as a working unit to help reduce sensitive or painful areas. Shoes for older adults can be selected and modified to support flexible deformities, accommodate fixed deformities, and control or limit motion as needed to compensate for degenerative joint changes that occur in the foot.

Shoes for older adults must protect and provide comfort as well as assist in both stance and locomotion to help them cope with the environmental changes in society: hard, flat surfaces or the plane of support; the social and psychologic pressures of society; and the effects of prolonged and repetitive microtrauma associated with occupational needs, the weight of the individual, and the effects of the shoes' last, construction, and material in relation to incompatibilities. It also is important to recognize the older adult as a human being who still wants to function as an integral member of society; the impact of disease and disability on shoe selection; and changes such as atrophy and hypertrophy, neuromuscular responses, or psychic or psychogenic responses, involving the individual as a whole.

ANATOMY OF A SHOE

The modern shoe is defined by the last, which determines the shape and cubical content of the shoe. The various forms of construction and materials will vary depending on the shoe's projected use and cost. The height of the heel may have a direct relationship to design, with men's shoes generally having a military, or lower, heel. Shoes that generally are defined as *orthopedic* usually have a Thomas heel, which provides an extension of the medial portion for the heel for additional support, but the use of the molded sole and wedge design provides footwear that essentially is unisex. See Figure 23 for an illustration of a shoe.

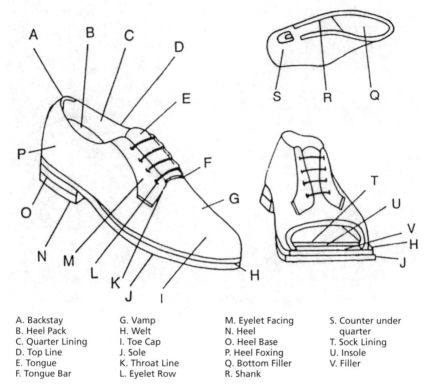

A. Backstay	G. Vamp	M. Eyelet Facing	S. Counter under
B. Heel Pack	H. Welt	N. Heel	quarter
C. Quarter Lining	I. Toe Cap	O. Heel Base	T. Sock Lining
D. Top Line	J. Sole	P. Heel Foxing	U. Insole
E. Tongue	K. Throat Line	Q. Bottom Filler	V. Filler
F. Tongue Bar	L. Eyelet Row	R. Shank	

Figure 23.   Components of a shoe. (From Pedorthic Footwear Association. [n.d.]. *Pedorthic reference guide.* Columbia, MD: Author. Copyright © Pedorthic Footwear Association, Columbia, MD, 1992, 1999, 2006. All rights reserved. Reprinted with permission.)

The upper of the shoe usually includes portions that are referred to as the vamp, quarter, lace stay, top facing, back stay, collar, linings, foxing, toe box, and shank piece and has such designations as the throat, shank, vamp line, and toe box depth. The vamp is the lower part of the upper that attaches to the sole or the welt. The quarter usually refers to the back portion, or heel area, of the upper, or the portion that would go around the outline of the counter. The lace stay usually refers to a reinforcement of leather or other material that is found in front of the insertion of the lace eyelets. The lace stay covers the tongue, which is a protective piece of leather or other material that provides protection of the foot from the eyelets and lacings. Many shoes have a padded collar to add to the comfort of footwear.

Better shoes generally have two linings for additional protection, but when they are broken or cracked, they can cause limited pressure points. The same is true for foxing or trimmings.

The box, or tip, of the shoe usually is reinforced over the toes, providing rigidity for additional protection and style. Very shallow toe boxes create compression incompatibilities, especially with digital contractures and edema. Higher toe boxes provide greater depth. The counter of the shoe by classic design is a rigid reinforcement for the heel area. A long counter extends the medial segment to the navicular area.

The insole, depending on the type of shoe construction and material used, provides the initial contact between the sole of the foot and other segments of the shoe, such as the sock lining, filler, counter under quarter, bottom filler, and shank, as well as the welt and the sole. The filler usually consists of ground cork between the insole. With molded soles, some of the traditional shoe construction is modified. The outsole is the portion of the shoe that is used for ground support.

The thickness and the selection of materials that compose the insole, outsole, and fillers have an effect on the weight-diffusive capacities of the shoe. Once worn for a period of time, the weight-dispersive qualities of the material are manifest from the effects of weight bearing, loading, and ambulation, in relation to the foot and its function.

The shank of the shoe usually refers to the area of the outsole between the breast of the heel and the widest portion of the outsole, when designating position. The shank piece is a rigid, supportive material (steel or laminate) that varies in width and determines the rigidity of the area on weight bearing. It is inserted in the heel center and the ball portion of the shoe. The shank pitch of the sole is the plane, or angle, of the shank area from the breast of the heel to the sole contact or ball of the foot. The modern wedge shoes and molded soles act in a sense as a shank filler and add rigidity. It should be noted that heel height, sole material, and shoe modifications are measured in eighths ($\frac{1}{8}''$).

Finally, an important part the geriatric shoe is its construction. Construction types include Goodyear welt, stitchdown, McKay, Littleway, turn sole, and molded sole. Shoe modification ease will depend on the type of construction.

Conditions that May Necessitate Shoe Modifications	
• Residuals of osteoarthritis	• Metatarsalgia
• Residuals of rheumatoid arthritis	• Intermetatarsal neuritis
• Hallux limitus	• Severe residual deformity
• Hallux rigidus	• Gouty arthritis
• Metatarsal phalangeal arthritis	• Calcaneal spur
• Amputated hallux	• Calcaneal bursitis
• Amputated digits	• Plantar fasciitis
• Hallux valgus, mild	• Limited dorsiflexion
• Hallux valgus, severe	• Peripheral vascular impairment
• Short first ray (Morton's syndrome)	• Limb length discrepancy, less than 1½″
• Hammertoes, digital contractures	• Limb length discrepancy, more than 1½″
• Flexible inverted heel	• Forefoot amputation, trans-metatarsal
• Flexible pes planus, mild or severe	• Forefoot amputation, Lisfranc or Chopart
• Rigid pes planus	• Charcot joint or foot
• Pes cavus, mild or rigid (severe)	• Unstable ankle

Sidebar 8

SHOE MODIFICATIONS

Shoe last needs to be compatible with foot types—for example, inflare, outflare, or straight—to compensate for foot shape. Where deformities exist, special lasts, such as bunion lasts or extra-depth lasts, may be needed.

When the older adult cannot be fit with a commercially available stock shoe, a depth, extra-depth, super-depth, or custom-molded shoe needs to be considered. Sidebar 8 lists examples of special needs that may necessitate shoe modifications.

Shoe modifications that commonly are used for the older adult include but are not limited to the following general concepts. The medial heel seat wedge is used for valgus deformities, and the lateral heel seat wedge is used for varus deformities that involve the heel. These wedges, placed between the heel and the outsole, sometimes are used with sole wedges to achieve gait modification and are used to provide better balance to the heel. Sole wedges usually are used with other shoe modifications (e.g., heel wedges) for alignment and support and to help attain a better gait pattern. The lateral sole wedge also may be called a *lateral Dutchman,* and all usually are placed between the outsole and the filler and adapted back into the welt.

The metatarsal bar is used to shift the weight from the metatarsal heads to locations along the metatarsal shafts. The bar is placed on the outsole as an external shoe modification and generally permit heel rise to push off without additional metatarsal head weight bearing. Bars usually are placed just proximal to the metatarsal heads. Modifications include the Denver bar (which may be placed internally); the Hauser bar, or comma bar; and other modifications of the principle.

The Thomas heel, a common component of the orthopedic shoe, is a medial extension of the heel to improve balance, provide additional support, and relieve pressure from the shank area. The heel may be reversed (reverse Thomas heel) to provide similar functions for the lateral aspect of the shoe.

A flared heel is used to provide broader support and additional stability to the ankle and the heel from rolling over. The flare may be used either medially or laterally. The extension of the flare usually is equal to the widest portion of the counter.

A shank filler, in effect, turns any shoe into a wedge shoe by filling in the area between the anterior portion of the heel and the contact point of the outsole. By filling in the area between the breast of the heel and the toe break, a total-contact weight-bearing area can be provided, and the shank area then becomes more stable. Shank filler also can be used medially for excessive valgus of the foot and laterally for excessive varus of the foot.

When there is a loss of push-off function in gait, a long steel stiffener that is extended to the toes can be used. It precludes the shoe from remaining in a dorsiflexed position. It usually is placed from the breast of the heel to the anterior toe area, between the outsole and the filler, as would be a steel shank. In a sense, it is a spring extension of the steel shank.

A rocker bar is a modification of the metatarsal bar and is designed to prevent flexion or extension of the shoe. It can be used where pain is present with toe bending. It functions during rocking of weight into heel rise and push off. The bar usually extends from the mid-shank area to just proximal to the anterior tip of the shoe, with the widest point of the shoe usually at the highest point of the rocker bar.

When there is a need to provide simulated plantar flexion (extension) or ankle motion, a solid ankle cushion heel, can be ordered. This provides a soft wedge at the posterior inferior tip of the heel of the shoe at heel strike. When there is some shortage of the extremity, a heel seat cushion can be added internally. When greater motion is desired and there is no clinical shortage of significance, adding a heel cushion to the opposite shoe will provide such response. Limiting motion with a solid ankle cushion heel can be accomplished by using a metatarsal bar, rocker bar, steel spring, or double sole. Heel stabilizers can be used to eliminate lateral forces that tend to turn the heel or the ankle, such as in postfracture care.

Long steel springs can be used to strengthen the shoe and reinforce the arch area of a lightweight shoe. The spring is placed at the center of the heel to the widest portion of the outsole, between the outsole and the filler or between the insole and the outsole. See Figure 24 for examples of shoe modifications.

When there are significant limb length problems, cork or other material build-ups can be fabricated. Neoprene crepe also can be used for this function as well as for shock absorption and weight diffusion. When modified properly, the same materials also can be adapted for

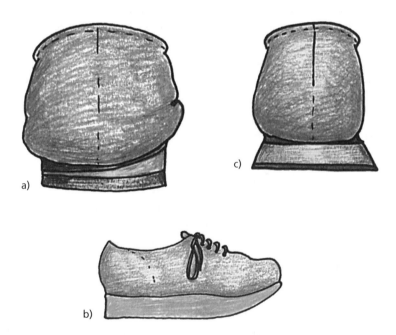

Figure 24. Examples of shoe modifications: a) lateral heel wedge, b) toe rocker sole, c) flared heel. (From Helfand, A.E. [1994]. *If the shoe fits* [pp. 4, 7, & 8]. Harrisburg, PA: Professional Diabetes Academy. Artwork by Ray Wherley. Reprinted with permission.)

weight dispersion. When there is significant limb length shortage that cannot be managed by these methods, a skate build-up or extension (i.e., platform addition to increase height) can be prescribed. Stability must be ensured to avoid ankle injury.

Various forms of shoe modification also have been used, such as adding the filler under metatarsal or calcaneal areas for pain. However, orthoses that are used properly are more effective and tend to be less costly for the individual because they can be transferred from shoe to shoe. Additional shoe modifications include medial longitudinal arch pads (or "cookies"), metatarsal pads, internal heel wedges, calcaneal bars, heel pads and lifts, and Barton and Thomas wedges.

Shoe modifications can be considered when shoe lasts are compatible with foot types, when shoe construction can be considered for modification, and when the individual will comply. Custom-molded shoes should be considered when therapeutic modifications cannot be completed in an efficient manner.

Shoe selection also needs to focus on the basic shoe types—bal, blucher, low cut, high top, and surgical—as well as the functional needs of the individual. When orthotics or other internal shoe modifications are to be considered, appropriate last must be used to accommodate for the depth reduction. Older adults generally are more comfortable with less rigidity and more flexibility unless specific deformities that require modification are present.

CONCLUSION

Footwear is needed for protection and should permit the individual to function as normally as possible. The shoe must function as a unit with the individual and be compatible with and supportive of the individual's functional requirements and ambulatory needs. Selection of shoes for older adults always should place comfort and function above style, but individuals also need to function in society, making intelligent compromise a consideration for the individual's overall welfare.

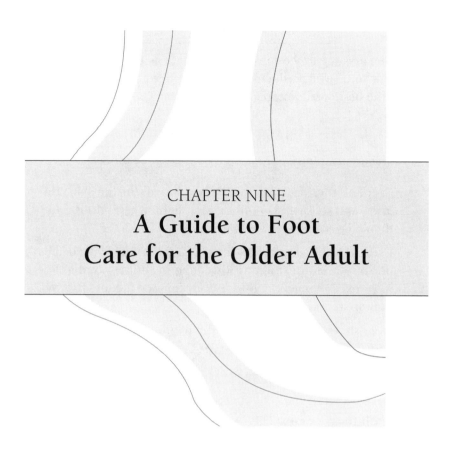

CHAPTER NINE

A Guide to Foot
Care for the Older Adult

M ost people take their feet for granted. Feet are vital to health and mobility, carrying a person thousands of miles in a lifetime. It is easy to understand why foot problems are common. As people age, these problems can get worse. To older adults, foot problems can mean the difference between needing institutional care and being able to live at home.

This chapter on proper foot care has been prepared for older adults but should be of interest to people of all ages who want to put their feet first. This chapter provides helpful suggestions for treating and preventing common foot problems. It is not intended, however, as a substitute for appropriate medical and podiatric care. If your feet hurt, then arrange to see a professional, such as a podiatrist, who will work with your primary doctor as well as other medical specialists to ensure the best possible care.

BASIC FOOT CARE

Following are simple steps to keep feet in good health:

- Examine the feet daily for dryness, breaks in the skin, calluses, and so forth. Do this in good light; if eyesight is poor, then have someone else do it.

- Use a moisturizing cream for dry and cracked skin. If feet perspire, then dust lightly with an appropriate powder. Remove excess cream or powder from between the toes to avoid skin breakdown.

- Wear shoes and socks that fit the feet and are comfortable, and change socks daily.

- Match the shoes to the activity.

- Exercise daily.

- Wash the feet every day. Always test the water temperature with a thermometer. The temperature should be approximately 92°F. If a thermometer is not available, then the wrist or the elbow can be used to test the temperature of the water to avoid burning the feet, particularly if circulation is poor. Pat—do not rub—feet dry, and be sure to dry between and under the toes.

- Trim or file normal nails straight across and never shorter than the end of the toe. Never cut into the corners of the toenails. Use nail clippers; scissors; a rounded, diamond-chip nail file; or an emery board. If vision, bending, or balancing is a problem or if a medical condition that is an at-risk indicator— such as diabetes, peripheral arterial disease, or some other condition that limits circulation and/or sensation—is present, then seek appropriate professional care.

See a doctor right away if any of the following is observed:

- An injury that does not heal or becomes infected

- Any part of the foot or the leg that turns blue or black

- Pain when walking that is relieved by rest

- Reduced sensation to pain or extreme temperatures

- Any unusual coldness, cramping, numbness, tingling, or discomfort in the feet

COMMON FOOT PROBLEMS

Diabetes and Poor Circulation

For a person who has diabetes or poor circulation, it is especially important to pamper the feet. Individuals with diabetes may have a higher risk for ulcers and infection, be slower to heal, and be prone to poor circulation. Signs of poor circulation, which often comes with aging and is common among smokers, are a blue or purplish skin color, weak or nonexistent pulses in the feet, and slow healing of cuts. Bleeding under a toenail without injury also is common and may be classified as a *splinter hemorrhage*. When these problems are not recognized and treated, they can lead to gangrene and amputation. For this reason, the following precautions should be taken:

- Check the feet daily for cuts, blisters, and cracks.

- Avoid all activities that decrease blood circulation, such as smoking and crossing the legs or ankles when sitting. In cold weather, dress warmly from head to toe, because chilling any part of the body decreases circulation.

- Do not use heating pads or hot water bottles because they may burn the feet.

- Wear proper footwear or specially prescribed footwear to protect the feet from injury.

- Do not wear tight shoes, socks, or stockings.

- Use elastic laces to allow the feet to swell and move freely.

- Exercise every day to improve circulation and keep the feet healthy.

Fungal Infection: Athlete's Foot

Athlete's foot is a chronic fungal infection that generally is found between the toes. The skin is white, peeling, and cracked and sometimes becomes itchy, red, moist, and secondarily infected by bacteria. If the condition persists, then consult a professional, who probably will prescribe antifungal medication. Keeping the feet clean and dry; wearing clean, roomy, soft, proper socks that are changed daily; and alternating shoes every other day all are helpful.

Plantar Warts

Warts are caused by a virus that enters the skin directly either at pressure points or where the foot has been injured. Sometimes these warts can be mistaken for ingrown calluses on the bottom of the feet. A wart usually is round and has a crater in the center. It is called *plantar* because it is on the plantar surface, or sole, of the foot. Consult a professional for advice on treatment, shoes, padding, dressing, medication, or surgical removal. Warts are not a do-it-yourself project. The foot can be painfully scarred from improper treatment.

Corns and Calluses

Corns and calluses are thickenings of the skin. These often are caused by foot deformities, imbalance, a lack of soft tissue, joint displacement, and arthritic changes that are subject to excessive pressure, and they may be related to incompatible or poorly fitting, improper shoes or tight socks. Corns generally form on toes, and calluses form on the bottom of the foot. Corns and calluses also can be caused by faulty weight bearing—that is, when the weight is not evenly distributed and excessive pressure is placed on an adjacent structure or the ball of the foot. Consult a professional for the treatment of corns and calluses. Specially fitted inserts can be effective, help absorb shock, and redistribute pressure. Do not trim or pare corns or calluses with scissors or razor blades or use corn remedies—including pads that contain acid, which can burn the skin around the corn. Home treatment should be limited to rubbing lightly with a moisturizing cream and using a foot powder to reduce friction when the foot is dry.

Ulcers

Ulcers of the feet are open sores that do not heal. People with diabetes or poor circulation are particularly prone to ulcers of the feet because their sense of pain and temperature in their feet is diminished. They develop insensitivity to excessive pressure and are not aware of the warning signs. Consult an appropriate health care professional for care.

Ingrown Toenails

An ingrown toenail is a painful condition that often is caused by poor self-care, toenail deformity, and excessive pressure. The nail grows into the skin, causing the toe to become red and swollen as a result of infection (Figure 25). Ingrown toenails must be treated by a health care professional. A segment or portion of the nail may have to be removed, and antibiotics may be required to manage any infection. To help prevent infection of ingrown toenails, trim or file nails straight across and never shorter than the end of the toe. File any rough edges because they can cut into the next toe and cause problems.

Thick or Enlarged Toenails and Loose Nails

There are many causes for an abnormal thickening of toenails—for example, aging, fungal infection, diabetes, peripheral arterial disease, trauma, and psoriasis. Thickened or enlarged toenails can cause pressure sores and restricted movement, especially in older adults and individuals with diabetes. Loose, detached nails sometimes are caused by ongoing fungus infection or associated with the ongoing skin condition psoriasis. Consult a professional for either of these conditions.

Strained Arches

Strained arches, sometimes called fallen arches, are common because of foot deformity; imbalance; and walking on hard, flat surfaces, such as cement and pavement. Arches do not truly fall. Imbalance causes muscle weakening and a rotation of foot structure with changes in

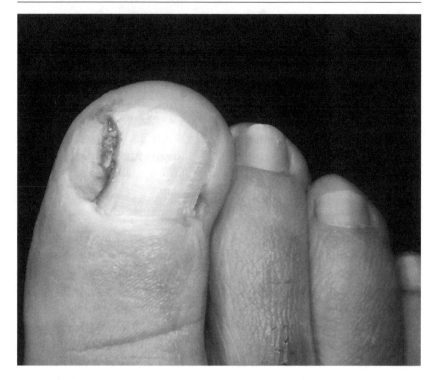

Figure 25. Infected ingrown toenail.

function. Symptoms are tired feet, pain in the legs, and low back pain. If any of these symptoms is present, then wear well-fitting, comfortable shoes that provide good support and do foot exercises. If the symptoms continue, then consult a professional. Special orthotics often relieve the condition. Physical modalities, such as whirlpool and exercise, coupled with other measures, also can provide relief.

Hammertoes

Hammertoes are caused by a muscle imbalance, possibly inherited; joint deformities that are associated with arthritis; or muscle wasting that is caused by a variety of systemic diseases. Wearing shoes that are too short, thereby causing the smaller toes to buckle, creates additional pressure that exaggerates the condition. The joints may stiffen permanently in this position. Corns form where the toes rub against the top of the shoes. If the pain persists, then consult a professional.

Wearing shoes with a high or deep toe box and a wider fit and using pads to ease the pressure both help. Special protective padding, silicone molds, and possibly surgery may be required in addition to the above measures.

Hallux Rigidus

Hallux rigidus is a type of joint deformity that is caused by an arthritis that involves the great toe joint. This joint between the great toe and the first metatarsal becomes stiff or completely immovable, often causing pain and limiting motion, making normal activities painful. Spurs develop around the joint, thereby producing a mechanical limitation of motion. Orthotics and special shoe modifications can help to reduce the pain and discomfort. The condition may require surgical joint revision and/or replacement for correction.

Metatarsalgia

Metatarsalgia refers to pain that is in the front of the foot and aggravated by abnormal pressure. It usually is associated with a high-arched foot or the spreading of the front of the foot with age. Pain also is associated with atrophy and displacement of the plantar fat pad, reducing the body's normal protective mechanism. It results in a dull burning and/or pain in the ball of the foot. Consult a professional for care if the pain persists.

Bunions

A bunion, or hallux valgus, usually is a painful deformity of the foot that consists of an enlargement at the inner side of the great toe joint and is caused when the great toe angles toward the second toe (Figures 26 and 27). Bunions, metatarsalgia, and hammertoes often occur together. Although a predisposition for bunions tends to be hereditary, they frequently are aggravated by biomechanical and pathomechanical changes in the foot. Patients are at greater risk as a result of improper and inappropriate footwear when they are young. Consult a professional, who may X-ray the feet and perform surgery to realign the bone or insert an artificial joint. Various shields and pads are available to relieve the pain of bunions and to hold the toe in alignment.

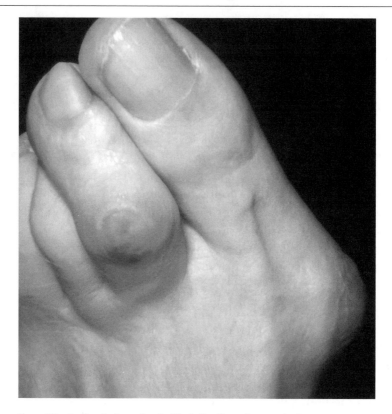

Figure 26. Bunion (hallux valgus) with digitus flexus (hammertoe).

Physical modalities, local steroids, and nonsteroidal anti-inflammatory drugs also may be used to reduce the pain and swelling. Wearing well-fitted shoes and socks or special bunion-lasted shoes may relieve the pain and discomfort of bunions. The bunion area of the shoe also can be stretched.

Heel Pain

Pain in the heel can be caused when the ligament-like structure that runs from the heel to the front of the foot is stretched and partially pulled away from its attachment to the heel. Consult a professional, who probably initially will order X-rays to rule out a heel spur and then physical therapy, orthotics, a plastic heel cup, or foam rubber padding in the shoe. A cortisone injection sometimes helps. To pre-

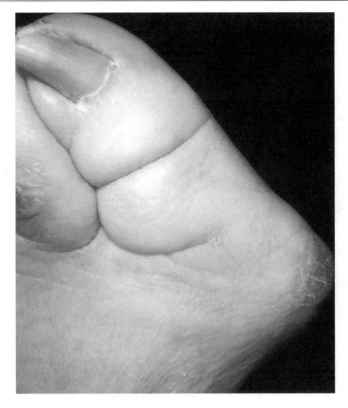

Figure 27. Bunion (hallux valgus).

vent this problem, wear comfortable, well-fitting shoes that provide good support.

Another painful condition in the heel is caused when the shoe rubs the bone at the back of the heel and becomes inflamed. An enlarged bursitis results and usually involves the heel cord, or Tendo Achilles. Padding and massaging the backs of new shoes to soften them before wearing them can prevent this.

Cracked heels, known as heel fissures, usually are caused by excessively dry and thickened skin and are related to excessive friction (Figure 28). A history of diabetes and peripheral arterial diseases contributes to their development. If heel cracks are painful, then consult a professional. At early signs of cracking, the heels can be rubbed with an appropriate emollient (cream or ointment).

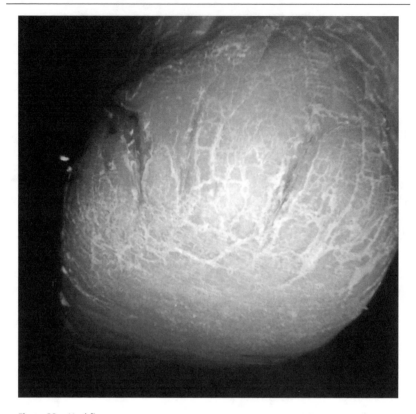

Figure 28. Heel fissures.

Fatigue or Stress Fractures

Fatigue or stress fractures usually are small fractures of a metatarsal bone (Figure 29). They often are a sign of abnormal weight bearing on an extra-long metatarsal bone, usually the second one. Under the stress, the bone cracks, causing swelling and pain. A professional can treat these fractures with immobilization and surgical shoes. Keeping as active as possible helps in the healing process.

Interdigital Neuroma

Pain in the front of the foot, especially when standing or walking, sometimes is due to swelling of a nerve, causing it to be pinched between the front ends of the metatarsal bones. Consult a professional. This sometimes can be relieved by an orthotic or a steroid injection. If

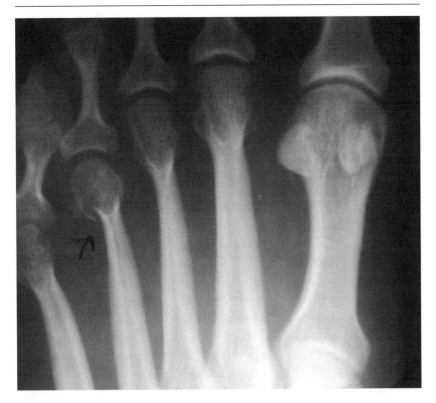

Figure 29.   Stress fracture (indicated by arrow).

the pain persists, then the swollen part of the nerve can be surgically removed.

Arthritis

The common types of arthritis in the feet are osteoarthritis, rheumatoid arthritis, and gout (which commonly involves the great toe joint). Osteoarthritis is due to wear and tear and occurs mainly in older people. Its symptoms include pain, stiffness, swelling, and a grinding sensation, particularly after prolonged activity. Rheumatoid arthritis can affect people of all ages and leads to pain and swelling in the joints as well as fatigue, fever, and loss of appetite. In gout, the joint of the great toe is red, swollen, and painful. People with arthritis in the feet also are prone to corns and calluses as a result of restricted movement and deformity of the joints in their feet. Consult a professional, who may prescribe medication, padding, specially molded inserts, or surgery. Wear comfortable, well-fitting footwear; lose weight if necessary; and rest during the day if possible.

TREATMENT

Most of the common foot problems described in this chapter will require some kind of treatment sooner or later. It is preferable that it be sooner for older people, whose circulation probably has slowed down and who could lose a foot or a leg as a result of an untreated infection in the foot.

A professional will identify the condition, and treatment will take one of the following forms: medication, orthotics, or surgery. Medication can be prescribed as a pill, an injection, or a cream. An orthotic is a supportive and/or corrective device that is inserted inside the shoe and individually molded to the foot. They are made of a variety of materials, such as plastic, leather, cork, foam, silicone, and sponge. Such inserts adjust the way the weight is distributed and make it possible for the individual to live comfortably with many of these foot conditions. Surgery sometimes is required to correct foot conditions.

Medicare provides coverage for specific foot care services. Coverage is greater when there are systemic risk diseases that reduce circulation and sensation to the feet, such as diabetes and peripheral arteriosclerosis (see Appendix).

FOOTWEAR

The foot tends to spread in the front under the body's weight as a person ages. Because most shoes are narrower in the front than the foot itself, shoes can contribute to a variety of problems. To determine whether a shoe is too narrow, put the foot down on a piece of paper and trace around the bottom, then compare the tracing with the shoe. If the foot is wider than the shoe, then it is time to go shopping for a new pair of shoes.

Proper Fit

Following are guidelines to ensure proper fit of shoes:

* Buy shoes at a good shoe store where experienced staff can help get the best fit.

- Shop late in the afternoon because feet swell during the day.

- Have both feet measured every time shoes are purchased, because one often is larger than the other. Try on both shoes, and buy them for the bigger foot.

- A properly fitting shoe should not touch the tips of the toes, cramp the width of the foot, or slip off the back of the heel. The toe box, or front of the shoe, should be roomy enough to allow the toes to move.

- Break in new shoes gradually to prevent blisters. Do not wear new shoes for more than 2 hours at a time, and, if necessary, protect sensitive parts of the feet with padding.

Good Construction

Following are guidelines to ensure that shoes are constructed well:

- Wear shoes that are appropriate for the activity: sturdy shoes with good support for walking; steel-toed boots for heavy work to protect feet from injury; jogging shoes for jogging; and warm, waterproof boots for winter.

- The upper part of the shoe should be firm enough to provide support, and the shoe should fasten securely.

- Heels should be a sensible height. A heel that is higher than 1¼″ (3 centimeters) throws the body's weight off center and leads to backaches and muscle cramps in the legs. If high heels must be worn, then switch heel heights during the day to ease strain on legs and feet.

- Leather is the best material because it is porous and can take the shape of the foot. Other materials, such as canvas and newer fabrics, can be used, provided that the shoes are worn for limited periods and for the activities for which they were designed.

- Insoles can be inserted in the shoe to absorb the jolts of walking.

- Soles should be strong and flexible and have a good gripping surface.

Care of Shoes

Shoes will be more comfortable when they are cared for properly.

- Polish new shoes before wearing them to increase their suppleness. Continue to polish frequently, and use saddle soap on leather shoes once a month.

- When shoes are not being worn, use shoetrees or shapers to keep them in shape.

- Keep shoes in good repair, replacing worn and broken-down heels, which weaken the ankles and cause balance problems.

- If soles are slippery, then improve traction by having a shoemaker put antislip material on the soles and heels of the shoes. Soles should be strong and flexible and have a good gripping surface.

FITNESS

Foot Exercises

Simple foot exercises help to maintain muscle tone, keep feet from getting tired, and protect against cramps. Here are some good exercises that can be done every day:

- While sitting down, lift a foot off the ground, hang a purse or small bag from the foot, and flex the foot to strengthen the ankle.

- Pick up marbles or a crumpled towel with toes.

- Rock in a rocking chair by pushing off with the toes.

- Stand with feet approximately 2″ apart and walk in a straight line with all of the weight on the outer edges of the feet.

- Rise on the balls of the feet and then rock back to the heels 20 times.

- Roll feet over a rolling pin several times a day.

- Cross legs, point the toe down, and move the foot in circles, first clockwise, then counterclockwise. The foot also can be rotated gently in and out and moved up and down at the ankle.

Walking: The Perfect Exercise

Walking is one of the best exercises for older people because it is not strenuous and costs nothing. Simply walking every day can

- Improve circulation and reduce the risk for blood clots
- Reduce the risk for heart disease and heart attack and generally increase the heart's efficiency
- Strengthen bones and improve muscle tone
- Help control body weight
- Reduce stress, anxiety, and depression
- Enable more clear and creative thinking

Other low-impact activities, such as swimming, golfing, cross-country skiing, snowshoeing, and skating, are beneficial to the whole body and, ultimately, the feet. Keep as active as possible, and enjoy the benefits of healthy feet.

CHAPTER TEN

Diagnostic and Therapeutic Considerations for Geriatricians

F oot problems in older adults are common and are major factors in podalgia, limitation of mobility, developmental functional disability, impairment, ambulatory dysfunction, gait imbalance, and increasing pain and discomfort. Foot impairments, changes, and deformities also present risk factors for the development of many significant complications of multiple systemic diseases and the potential for lower extremity amputation. Through the course of one's lifetime, the foot undergoes a great deal of trauma, use, misuse, and neglect. The stress of normal activity, changes that are associated with the aging process, systemic diseases, focal impairment, and environmental factors that are associated with ambulation create discomfort that can change the individual's ability to function as an independent

Table 4. Sample outline for the examination and recording of foot health data

Vascular
Posterior tibial pulse
Dorsalis pedis pulse
Popliteal pulse
Femoral pulse
Doppler studies
Edema
Calf tenderness

Integument

Toenails	*Skin*
Onychauxis	Color
Hypertrophy	Moisture
Onychogryphosis	Temperature
Incurvation	Texture
Deformity	Interspaces
Onychocryptosis	Fissures
Onychophosis	Ulcers
Onychomycosis	Tinea
Onycholysis	Tyloma
Onychomadesis	Heloma
Onychopathy	Xerosis
Onychia	Dermopathy
Paronychia	Atrophy
Subungual heloma	
Onychorrhexis	

Neurological
Achilles reflex
Patellar reflex
Superficial plantar
  reflex
Vibratory
Proprioception
Pain
Temperature

Musculoskeletal

Deformities	*Gait evaluation*	*Strength*	*Atrophy*
Hallux valgus	Foot type	Dorsiflexors	Foot
Hammertoes	Heel to toe	Plantarflexors	Leg
Spurs	Eversion	Invertors	
Rotations	Inversion	Evertors	
Varus and valgus deformities	Foot structural change		
Neurotrophic arthropathy	Ambulation aids		

member of society and that can generate additional psychological correlates.

PODIATRIC ASSESSMENT

The assessment, evaluation, and examination of the older adult in relation to his or her podiatric or foot health concerns involves more than the clinical knowledge of the foot and its demonstrated symptoms and signs. It is important to recognize the individual's concerns and needs in relation to pain, limitation of walking, and a special concern for comfort. Attention to primary goals, such as to relieve pain, restore the individual to a maximum level of function, and maintain that function once achieved, is the primary focus for care. The practitioner must anticipate projected changes that relate to ambulation and foot care needs and ensure individual dignity.

Table 4 is a sample outline for the examination and recording of foot health data. The initial element of the assessment should include the demographic data of the patient and his or her living conditions and then move on to foot complaints. Foot complaints and/or conditions need to be considered as

Conditions that Can Produce Foot Problems	
• Diabetes	• Mental retardation
• Arteriosclerosis	
• Ischemia	• Cerebral vascular accidents/stroke
• Buerger's disease	
• Chronic thrombophlebitis	• Transient ischemic attacks
• Venous stasis	• Thyroid disease
• Peripheral neuropathies	• Milroy's disease
• Malnutrition	• Anticoagulation therapy
• Alcohol abuse	• Hemiparesis or quadriparesis
• Chemical/substance abuse	
• Malabsorption	• Ventilator dependence
• Pernicious anemia	• Rayland's disease/syndrome
• Anemia	• Vitamin deficiencies
• Hemophilia	
• Cancer	• Osteoarthritis
• Drug interactions	• Rheumatoid arthritis
• Toxic states	• Gout
• Multiple sclerosis	• Obesity
• Uremia	• Psoriasis
• Chronic renal disease	• Urticaria
• Chronic obstructive pulmonary disease	• Atopic dermatitis
	• Pruritus
• Coronary artery disease	• Hyperhidrosis
	• Localized neurodermatitis
• Congestive heart failure	• Hysterical paralysis
• Hypertension	• Psychogenic tremors
• Edema	• Parkinson's disease
• Posttrauma	
• Leprosy	• Functional disability
• Neurosyphilis	
• Hereditary disorders/diseases	• Ambulatory dysfunction
• Mental illness	

Sidebar 9

Clinical Findings of Hyperkeratosis and Onychial and Dermatologic Lesions to Record as Signs of Disease, Deformity, and/or Disorder

- Dryness of the skin
- Xerosis
- Chronic tinea pedis
- Keratotic lesions
- Subkeratotic hemorrhage (plantar and digital)
- Trophic ulcerations
- Pressure ulcerations
- Diminished or absent hair growth
- Trophic nail changes (onychopathy)
- Onychogryphosis (ram's horn nail)
- Onychauxis (hypertrophic and thickened nails)
- Onychomycosis (fungal nails)
- Onychophosis (callused nail grooves)
- Hypertrophic deformity
- Subungual hemorrhage
- Ulceration (disease complication)
- Abscess
- Ingrown toenail (onychocryptosis)
- Onychia (inflammation)
- Paronychia (infection and inflammation)
- Incurvated or involuted toenails
- Foot type
- Gait
- Postural deformities
- Palpation of pain
- Range of motion
- Angulation
- Frank deformities (cavus feet, drop foot, hallux valgus, digiti flexus [hammertoes])
- Arthropathy (the pedal vasculature and related structures should be evaluated)

Sidebar 10

they relate to both activities of daily living (e.g., ambulation, dressing, grooming, bathing) and instrumental activities of daily living (e.g., shopping, housekeeping, transportation). The chief complaint of the patient should be explored in the patient's own terms and should include an exploration of the patient's perception of his or her condition and how the foot problems affect his or her daily life and activities. Footwear should be assessed in relation to fit, function, use, and compatibility with foot type and ambulatory use. The present condition should be noted as to duration, location, severity, previous treatment, and results and in relation to other general medical conditions.

A systems review should be completed along with a notation of other practitioners of record. Current medications and responses should be identified in relation to current and past therapeutic programs. The medical history should include infections, operations, fractures, injuries, and drug sensitivities and allergies. In addition, notation should be made of problems and diseases that have pedal complications and/or affect care and ambulation. See Sidebar 9 for examples of such risk conditions as delineated in Medicare regulations.

A review of the patient's podiatric history and foot care history should be noted as well as elements of self-care and the use of commercial foot care products. The occupational history should be explored and include foot/work-related activities, exposure, military service, geographic location, percentage of weight bearing, flooring, and footwear. The social history should include the use of tea, alcohol, coffee, and tobacco; sleeping habits; sedative and/or hypnotic use; use of narcotics and other drugs; and the reaction of the patient to his or her own illness or condition.

The subjective symptoms should be noted clearly as described by the patient and should attempt to focus, for example, on the following:

Dermatological

- Intensely painful or painless lesions
- Slow-healing or nonhealing wounds or necrosis
- Skin color changes such as cyanosis or redness
- Chronic itching, scaling, or dry feet
- Recurrent infections such as paronychia, athlete's foot, fungal toenails, and so forth

Peripheral vascular

- Cold feet
- Intermittent claudication involving the calf or the foot
- Pain at rest, especially nocturnal, relieved by dangling the feet or standing

Musculoskeletal

- Gradual change in foot shape
- Change in shoe size
- Painless change in foot shape
- Ambulatory dysfunction
- Joint changes and deformity

Neurological

- Sensory change
- Burning

- Tingling

- Clawing sensation

- Motor changes

- Weakness

- Foot drop

- Autonomic changes, such as diminished sweating

Clinical findings of hyperkeratosis and onychial and dermatologic lesions should be recorded as signs of disease, deformity, and/or a disorder. See Sidebar 10 for examples. Findings and/or conditions that allow Medicare to provide payment for primary foot care should be identified (see Appendix—Class Findings).

Absent popliteal or femoral pulses, bruits, dependent rubor with plantar pallor on elevation, and prolonged capillary filling time (> 3–4 seconds) should be recorded. Arterial skin temperature and blood pressure should be noted. Doppler studies, pulse volume recordings, and oscillometric readings also may be useful. Radiographic studies should be obtained as indicated and may include weight- and non–weight-bearing comparisons.

The neurological elements should include gait review, reflexes (patellar, Achilles, and superficial plantar), ankle clonus, vibratory sense, weakness, sensory deficits (proprioception, pain, and temperature perception), hyperesthesia, and autonomic dysfunction. The drug history should focus on but not be limited to antihypertensives, antidiabetics, cortisone, sedatives, topicals, antibiotics, antiarthritics, and other related medications that are used for and by older adults. The use of over-the-counter foot care remedies, including caustic foot keratotic applications, should be explored.

Some of the conditions that precipitate pain and discomfort in older adults and are related to functional imbalance and dysfunction include, for example the following:

- Pes planus

- Pes valgo planus

- Plantar imbalance

- Prolapsed metatarsal heads

- Fasciitis
- Myofasciitis
- Tendonitis
- Myositis
- Hallux valgus
- Hallux abducto valgus
- Digiti flexus
- Digital and phalangeal rotational deformities
- Hyperostosis
- Exostosis
- Spur formation
- Calcaneal spurs
- Bursitis
- Fibrositis
- Neuritis
- Neuroma
- Morton's syndrome
- Soft tissue atrophy
- Enthesopathy
- Hallux limitus
- Hallux rigidus
- Varus and valgus deformities of both the anterior and posterior segments of the foot

The pedal manifestations of diabetes in the older adult involve multiple systems and are associated with a variety of symptoms and signs, such as the following:

- Paresthesia
- Sensory impairment
- Motor weakness

- Reflex loss
- Neurotrophic arthropathy
- Muscle atrophy
- Dermopathy
- Onychopathy
- Absent pedal pulses
- Ischemia
- Trophic changes
- Neurotrophic ulceration
- Angiopathy
- Neuropathy
- Infection
- Necrosis and gangrene

Peripheral arterial insufficiency is present to some degree in many older adults. Overt indications of decreased arterial supply include, for example, the following:

- Muscle fatigue
- Cramps
- Claudication
- Pain
- Coldness
- Pallor
- Paresthesia
- Burning
- Atrophy of soft tissue
- Muscle wasting
- Trophic skin changes
- Dryness

- Hair loss
- Absent pedal pulses
- Calcification noted radiographically
- Edema

LONG-TERM CARE

The Standards for Long Term Care as developed by the Joint Commission on Accreditation of Healthcare Organizations include foot health and care as quality assurance issues. A similar component is being instituted for the current revision to the Medicare and Medicaid conditions of participation for long-term care facilities. These documents suggest as a basic consideration administrative projections to ensure foot health and care for the individual per the following guidelines:

Foot care and/or podiatric services are organized and staffed in a manner that is designed to meet the foot health needs of patient/residents.

The facility's foot health services should be provided by a podiatrist or appropriately licensed practitioner with a podiatric practitioner as a consultant.

A foot health program should be an integral part of the facility's total health care program.

Written policies and procedures should be developed to serve as a guide to the provision of podiatric/foot care services.

The consulting or supervising podiatrist participates in patient/resident care management as appropriate.

The quality and the appropriateness of podiatric services are monitored as an integral part of the overall quality assurance program, consistent with other practitioner/professional services.

CONTINUING EDUCATION

A program of professional, in-service, and patient education should be part of a total geriatric program. See Table 5 for a projected educational outline.

Table 5.   Outline of sample program for professional, in-service, and patient education

  I.   Relationship of foot problems to the older adult as a whole
       A.   Needs
       B.   Ambulation and independence
       C.   Diseases that put the individual at risk for problems
       D.   Factors that modify foot and health care in society
            1.   Medicare and Medicaid
       E.   Mental health considerations
       F.   Long-term care
       G.   Rehabilitation
 II.   Primary foot care
       A.   Assessment and examination
       B.   Nail disorders
       C.   Skin disorders
       D.   Hyperkeratotic disorders
       E.   Foot orthopedic and biomechanical (pathomechanical) changes
       F.   Foot deformities associated with aging
       G.   Diseases that put an older person at risk for foot problems
            1.   Diabetes mellitus
            2.   Arthritis
            3.   Gout
            4.   Vascular insufficiency
            5.   Other
       H.   Management
       I.   Interdisciplinary considerations
III.   Foot health education
       A.   Professional and interdisciplinary
       B.   Patient
IV.   Care delivery
       A.   Ambulatory care
       B.   Acute hospital considerations
       C.   Rehabilitation
       D.   Long-term care
       E.   Home care
       F.   Mental health issues and mental retardation
 V.   Interdisciplinary education
VI.   Footwear and related considerations

CONCLUSION

Given the high prevalence of foot problems in older adults, especially in those with chronic diseases and mental health problems, foot care needs are essential. Foot health, foot care, and foot health promotion should be part of comprehensive health care for older adults. The ability to remain active and ambulatory is one means of ensuring dignity and self-esteem for older adults.

Bibliography

Alexander, I.J. (1997). *The foot: Examination and diagnosis* (2nd ed.). New York: Churchill Livingstone.

American College of Foot and Ankle Surgeons. (2000). *Diabetic foot disorders: A clinical practice guideline.* Park Ridge, IL: Author.

American Diabetes Association. (1999). Consensus development conference on diabetic foot wound care. *Diabetes Care, 22*(8), 1354–1360.

American Diabetes Association. (2003). Preventive foot care in people with diabetes. *Diabetes Care, 26*(Suppl. 1), S78–S79.

American Podiatric Medical Association. (1977). *Foot health training: Guide for long term care personnel.* Washington, DC: Author.

Baran, R., Dawber, R.P.R., Tosti, A., & Haneke, E. (1996). *A text atlas of nail disorders, diagnosis, and treatment.* St. Louis: Mosby.

Baran, R., Hay, R., Haneke, E., Tosti, A. (1999). *Onychomycosis: The current approach to diagnosis and therapy.* London: Martin Dunitz.

Beaven, D.W., & Brooks, S.E. (1984). *Color atlas of the nail in clinical diagnosis.* Chicago: Year Book Medical Publishers.

Benvenuti, F., Ferrucci, L., Guralnik, J.M., Gangemi, S., & Baroni, A. (1995). Foot pain and disability in older persons: An epidemiologic survey. *Journal of the American Geriatrics Society, 43,* 479–484.

Bild, D.E., Selby, J.V., Sinnock, P., Browner, W.S., Braveman, P., & Showstack, J.A. (1989). Lower extremity amputation in people with diabetes: Epidemiology and prevention. *Diabetes Care, 12*(1), 23–31.

Birrer, R.B., Dellacorte, M.P., & Grisafi, P.J. (1988). *Common foot problems in primary care* (2nd ed.). Philadelphia: Henley & Belfus.

Bolton, A.J.M., Connor, H., & Cavanagh, P.R. (2000). *The foot in diabetes* (3rd ed.). New York: John Wiley & Sons.

Bottomley, J.M., & Lewis, C.B. (2003). *Geriatric rehabilitation: A clinical approach.* Upper Saddle River, NJ: Prentice Hall.

Bowker, J.H., & Pfeifer, M.A. (2001). *Levin's and Oneal's the diabetic foot* (6th ed.). St. Louis: Mosby.

Brachman, P.R. (1966). *Foot orthopedics.* Chicago: Interstate Printers and Publishers.

Brachman, P.R. (1966). *Mechanical foot therapy.* Chicago: Interstate Printers and Publishers.

Brachman, P.R. (1979). *Shoe therapy.* Chicago: Illinois College of Podiatric Medicine.

Brenner, M.A. (1987). *Management of the diabetic foot.* Baltimore: Lippincott Williams & Wilkins.

Brodie, B.S. (2001). Health determinants and podiatry. *Journal of the Royal Society for the Promotion of Health, 121*(3), 174–176.

Brody, S.J., & Pawlson, L.G. (1990). *Aging and rehabilitation II: The state of the practice.* New York: Springer Publishing Co.

Bryant, J.L., & Beinlich, N.R. (1999). Foot care: Focus on the elderly. *Orthopedic Nursing, 18*(6), 53–60.

Burns, A., Nitin, P., & Craig, S. (2002). *Mental health in older people.* London: Royal Society of Medicine Press.

Burns, S.L. (2002). Older people and ill-fitting shoes. *Postgraduate Medical Journal, 78*(920), 344–346.

Calkins, E., Davis, P.J., & Ford, A.B. (Eds.). (1986). *The practice of geriatrics.* Philadelphia: W.B. Saunders.

Cailliet, R. (1997). *Foot and ankle pain* (3rd ed.). Philadelphia: F.A. Davis Co.

Carleton, F.J. (1949). *Shoes and feet.* New York: New York Printing.

Cavanagh, P.R., Boone E.Y., & Plummer, D.L. (2000). *The foot in diabetes: A bibliography.* State College: Pennsylvania State University.

Centers for Medicare & Medicaid Services. (2002, March 27). *Program manual: Foot care and supportive devices for feet* (Chapter H, Section 2323). Baltimore: Social Security Administration.

Centers for Medicare & Medicaid Services. (2002, July 17). *Transmittal AB-02-096: Coverage and billing of the diagnosis and treatment of peripheral neuropathy with loss of protective sensation in people with diabetes.* Baltimore: Social Security Administration.

Collet, B.S. (2000). Foot disorders. In B.H. Beers & R. Berkow (Eds.), *The Merck manual of geriatrics* (17th ed.). Rathway, NJ: Merck Research Laboratories.

Crawford, L.S., Ahford, R.L., McPeake, B., & Stout, R.W. (1995). Conservative podiatric medicine and disability in elderly people. *Journal of the American Podiatric Medical Association, 85*(5), 255–259.

Dauber, R., Bristow, I., & Turner, W. (2001). *Text atlas of podiatric dermatology.* London: Martin Dunitz.

Dawson, J. (2002). The prevalence of foot problems in older women: A cause for concern. *Journal of Public Health Medicine, 24*(2), 77–84.

Eng, W. (1986–1987). Geriatric podiatry. In *Geriatric curriculum resource guides for health professionals* (p. 1). Richmond, VA: Geriatric Education Center at Virginia Commonwealth University.

Evans, J.G., Williams, T.F., Michel, J.-P., & Beattie, B. (2000). *Oxford textbook of geriatric medicine* (2nd ed.). New York: Oxford University Press.

Finucane, P., & Sinclair, A.J. (1995). *Diabetes in old age.* New York: John Wiley & Sons.

Frykberg, R.G. (1991). *The high risk foot in diabetes mellitus.* New York: Churchill Livingstone.

Gable, L.L. (Ed.), & Haines, D.J., & Papp, K.K. (Asst. Eds.). (2004). *The aging foot: An interdisciplinary perspective.* Columbus: The Ohio State University, College of Medicine and Public Health, Department of Family Medicine.

Guralnik, J.M., Ferrucci, L., Pieper, C.F., Leveille, S.G., Markides, K.S., Ostir, G.V., et al. (2000). Lower extremity function and subsequent disability: Consistency across studies, predictive models, and value of gait speed alone compared with the short physical performance battery. *The Journals of Gerontology. Series A, Biological Sciences and Medical Sciences, 55,* M221–M231.

Hack, N. (1989). *Fitting shoes.* Alexandria, VA: American Diabetes Association.

Harkless, L.B., & Krych, S.M. (1990). *Handbook of common foot problems.* New York: Churchill Livingtone.

Helfand, A.E. (1967). Podiatry in a total geriatric health program: Common foot problems of the aged. *Journal of the American Geriatrics Society, 15*(6), 593–599.

Helfand, A.E. (1968). Keep them walking. *Journal of the American Podiatric Medical Association, 58*(3), 117–126.

Helfand, A.E. (1969). The foot of South Mountain: A foot health survey of the residents of a state geriatric institution. *Journal of the American Podiatry Association, 59*(4), 133–139.

Helfand, A.E. (Ed.). (1981). *Clinical podogeriatrics.* Baltimore: Lippincott Williams & Wilkins.

Helfand, A.E. (1984). Basic considerations for shoes, shoes modifications, and orthoses in foot care. *Clinics in Podiatry, 1,*(2), 431–440.

Helfand, A.E. (Ed.). (1987). *Public health and podiatric medicine.* Baltimore: Lippincott Williams & Wilkins.

Helfand, A.E. (1990). Limiting mobility loss from foot problems. In S.J. Brody & L.G. Pawlson (Eds.), *Aging and rehabilitation: II—The state of the practice* (pp. 95–109). New York: Springer Publishing Co.

Helfand, A.E. (1993). Geriatric overview: Part I. *The Foot, 3,* 58–61.

Helfand, A.E. (Ed.). (1993). The geriatric patient and considerations of aging. *Clinics in podiatric medicine and surgery: Vol. 1.* Philadelphia: W.B. Saunders.

Helfand, A.E. (Ed.). (1993). The geriatric patient and considerations of aging. *Clinics in podiatric medicine and surgery: Vol. 2.* Philadelphia: W.B. Saunders.

Helfand, A.E. (1994). *If the shoe fits.* Harrisburg, PA: Professional Diabetes Academy.

Helfand, A.E. (1995). *Feet first.* Harrisburg: Pennsylvania Diabetes Academy.

Helfand, A.E. (1995). Geriatric overview: Part II. *The Foot, 5,* 19–23.

Helfand, A.E. (1996). What you need to know about therapeutic footwear. *Practical Diabetology, 15*(4), 4–9.

Helfand, A.E. (1998). *If the shoe fits.* Harrisburg: Pennsylvania Diabetes Academy.

Helfand, A.E. (1999). Podiatric services in long-term care. *Focus on Geriatric Care and Rehabilitation, 18*(4), 1–12.

Helfand, A.E. (1999). Public health strategies to develop a comprehensive chronic disease and podogeriatric protocol. *National Academies of Practice Forum, 1*(1), 49–57.

Helfand, A.E. (2000). A conceptual model for a geriatric syllabus for podiatric medicine. *Journal of the American Podiatric Medical Association, 90*(5), 258–267.

Helfand, A.E. (2001). *Assessing the older diabetic patient* [CD]. Harrisburg: Pennsylvania Diabetes Academy, Pennsylvania Department of Health, Temple University School of Medicine, Office for Continuing Medical Education, Temple University School of Podiatric Medicine.

Helfand, A.E. (2003). Clinical podogeriatrics: Assessment, education, and prevention. *Clinics in Podiatric Medicine and Surgery, 20*(3), xvii–xxiii.

Helfand, A.E. (2003). Diabetic foot: Assessment, management, and prevention. In B.J. Goldstein & D. Muller-Wieland (Eds.), *Textbook of type 2 diabetes* (pp. 255–273). London: Martin Dunitz.

Helfand, A.E. (2004). Clinical assessment of podogeriatric patients. *Podiatry Management, 23*(2), 145–152.

Helfand, A.E. (2004). Foot problems in older patients: A focused podogeriatric assessment study in ambulatory care. *Journal of the American Podiatric Medical Association, 94,*(3), 293–304.

Helfand, A.E. (2006). Diseases and disorders of the foot. In P. Pompei & J.B. Murphy (Eds.), *Geriatric review syllabus: A core curriculum in geriatric medicine* (6th ed., pp. 451–458). New York: American Geriatrics Society.

Helfand, A.E. (2006). *Diseases and disorders of the foot: Geriatric review syllabus* (5th ed.) [Slide Presentation]. New York: American Geriatrics Society.

Helfand, A.E., & Bruno, J. (Eds.). (1984). *Rehabilitation of the foot. Clinics in Podiatry: Vol. 1, No. 2.* Philadelphia: W.B. Saunders.

Helfand, A.E., Cooke, H.L., Walinsky, M.D., & Demp, P.H. (1998). Foot problems associated with older patients: A focused podogeriatric study. *Journal of the American Podiatric Medical Association, 88*(4), 237–241.

Helfand, A.E., & Jessett, D.F. (1998). Foot problems. In M.S.J. Pathy (Ed.). *Principles and practice of geriatric medicine* (3rd ed., pp. 1165–1176). New York: John Wiley & Sons.

Helfand, A.E., & Jessett, D.F. (2006). Foot problems in the elderly. In P.S. Pathy, A.J. Sinclair, & J.E. Morley (Eds.), *Principles and practice of geriatric medicine.* (4th ed., pp. 1311–1328). New York: John Wiley & Sons.

Highmark Government Services. (2002, June 2). *Medicare report: Coverage requirements for routine foot care* (pp. 33–36). Camp Hill, PA: Author.

Jahss, M.H. (Ed.). (1982). *Diseases of the foot.* Philadelphia: W.B. Saunders.

Jessett, D.F., & Helfand, A.E. (1991). Foot problems in the elderly. In M.S.J. Pathy (Ed.), *Principles and practice of geriatric medicine* (2nd ed., pp. 1301–1307). New York: John Wiley & Sons.

Klenerman, L. (Ed.). (1991). *The foot and its disorders* (3rd ed.). London: Blackwell Scientific Publications.

Kozak, G.P., Campbell, D.R., Frykberg, R.G., & Habershaw, G.M. (Eds.). *Management of diabetic foot problems* (2nd ed.). Philadelphia: W.B. Saunders.

Levy, L., & Hetherington, V. (Eds.). (2006). *Foot problems associated with aging: Principles and practice of podiatric medicine* (2nd ed.). Brooklandville, MD: Data-Trace Publishing Co.

Libow, L.B., & Sherman, F.T. (Eds.). (1981). *The core of geriatric medicine.* St. Louis: Mosby.

Lorimer, D., French, G., O'Donnell, M., & Burrow, J.G. (2002). *Neale's disorders of the foot: Diagnosis and management* (6th ed.). New York: Churchill Livingstone.

McCarthy, D.J. (Ed.). (1986). *Podiatric dermatology.* Baltimore: Lippincott Williams & Wilkins.

Merrill, H.E., Frankson, J., Jr., & Tarara, E.L. (1967). Podiatry survey of 1011 nursing home patients in Minnesota. *Journal of the American Podiatric Medical Association, 57* 57–64.

Merriman, L.M., & Tollafield, D.R. (1995). *Assessment of the lower limb.* New York: Churchill Livingstone.

Merriman, L.M., & Turner, W. (2002). *Assessment of the lower limb* (2nd ed.). New York: Churchill Livingstone.

National Diabetes Education Program. (n.d.). *Feet can last a lifetime: A health care provider's guide to preventing diabetes foot problems.* Retrieved June 5, 2006, from http://www.ndep.nih.gov/resources/feet/index.htm

Pedorthic Footwear Association. (n.d.). *Pedorthic reference guide.* Columbia, MD: Author.

Plummer, E.S., & Albert, S.G. (1996). Focused assessment of foot care in older adults. *Journal of the American Geriatrics Society, 44*(3), 310–313.

Reichel, W. (Ed.). (1989). *Clinical aspects of aging* (3rd ed.). Baltimore: Lippincott Williams & Wilkins.

Robbins, J.M. (1994). *Primary podiatric medicine.* Philadelphia: W.B. Saunders.

Rossi, W.A. (2000). *The complete footwear dictionary* (2nd ed.). Malabar, FL: Kreiger Publishing Co.

Rutherford, R.B., Baker, J.D., Ernest, C., Johnston, K.W., Porter, J.M., Ahn, S., & Jones, D.N. (1997). Recommended standards for reports dealing with lower extremity ischemia: Revised version. *Journal of Vascular Surgery, 26*(3), 517–538.

Samitz, M.H. (1981). *Cutaneous disorders of the lower extremities* (2nd ed.). Baltimore: Lippincott Williams & Wilkins.

Samman, P.D., & Fenton, D.A. (1986). *The nails in disease* (4th ed.) London: William Heinemann Medical Books.

Sims, D.S., Cavanagh, P., & Ulbrecht, J.S. (1988). Risk factors in the diabetic foot: Recognition and management. *Physical Therapy, 68,* 1887–1902.

Starin, I., & Kuo, N. (1966). The Queensbridge health maintenance service for the elderly, 1961–1965. *Public Health Reports, 81*(1), 75–82.

Strauss, M.B., Hart, J.D., & Winant, D.M. (1998). Preventive foot care. *Postgraduate Medicine, 103*(5), 233–245.

Tollafield, D.R., & Merriman, L.M. (1997). *Clinical skills in treating the foot.* New York: Churchill Livingstone.

Turner, W., & Merriman, L.M. (2005). *Clinical skills in treating the foot* (2nd ed.). New York: Churchill Livingstone.

U.S. Department of Health and Human Services. (2005, August). *Talking with your doctor* [NIH Publication No. 05-3452]. Bethesda, MD: National Institutes of Health, National Institute on Aging

U.S. Department of Veterans Affairs. (1984, August 10). *Podiatric medicine service, nursing home care units: Program guide M-2, part 1, G-1, 3.13.* Washington, DC: Author.

U.S. Department of Veterans Affairs. (2004, October 6). *Footwear and orthoses* [VHA Handbook 1173.9]. Washington, DC: Veterans Health Administration.

Williams, T.F. (Ed.). (1984). *Rehabilitation in the aging.* New York: Raven Press.

Witkowski, J.A. (Ed.). (1983). Diseases of the lower extremities. *Clinics in Dermatology: Vol. 1, No. 1.*(1). Baltimore: Lippincott Williams & Wilkins.

Woodside, N., & Shapiro, J. (1967). Podiatry service and clinics in a local health department. Experiences of the District of Columbia. *Public Health Reports, 82*(5), 389–394.

Yale, I., & Yale, J.F. (1984). *The arthritic foot and related connective tissue disorders.* Baltimore: Lippincott Williams & Wilkins.

Yale, J.F. (1987). *Yale's podiatric medicine* (3rd ed.). Baltimore: Lippincott Williams & Wilkins.

Glossary

TERMS THAT DENOTE LOCATION

anterior   Situated in front of or as the forward part of the body.

distal   Farthest from any point of reference (as opposed to proximal).

dorsum   The top surface of the foot.

inferior   Situated below; a structure that occupies the lowest position.

lateral   Side; a position away from the midline of the body.

medial   Middle; closer to the midline of the body.

plantar   Pertaining to the sole of the foot.

posterior   Situated in back of or as the back part of the body.

proximal   Nearest or closest to any point of reference (as opposed to distal).

superior   Situated above; a structure that occupies a higher position.

ANATOMIC DEFINITIONS

artery   Tubular vessel that carries the blood from the heart to other parts of the body.

bone   The substance that makes up the skeletal framework; gives the body form and rigidity.

ligament   Fibrous band of tissue that connects bone.

muscle   Organ attached to the bones that, by contracting, provides movement of the body.

nerve   Cord-like structure that conveys impulses between the brain and the central nervous system to other parts of the body.

tendon   Fibrous band of tissue that connects the muscles to the bones.

vein   Tubular vessel that carries the blood from other parts of the body back to the heart.

OTHER TERMS

abduction   To move away from a center line (as though it is drawn between the feet).

abscess   Localized collection of pus in a cavity.

Achilles tendon   A tendon that is attached to the posterior of the calcaneus and flexes the foot.

acromegaly   Hyperfunction of the eosinophilic cells of the anterior lobe of the pituitary gland with progressive overgrowth of bone.

adduction   To move toward a center line (as though it is drawn between the feet).

adhesion   Fibrous connection between two structures, whether soft tissue or hard, that may be a result of surgery, trauma, or infection.

amputation   The partial or total removal of an extremity.

amyotrophic lateral sclerosis (ALS)   A neurological syndrome marked by muscular weakness and atrophy with spasticity and hyperreflexia as a result of degeneration of the motor neurons of the spinal cord, medulla, and cortex; sometimes called Lou Gehrig's disease.

anatomy   Science of the structure of the body and relation of its parts.

anesthesia   Induced loss of feeling or sensation to permit surgery or other painful procedures.

antibiotic   Chemical substance with the ability to inhibit the growth of or to destroy bacteria and other microorganisms.

antiseptic   Substance that will inhibit the growth and development of microorganisms without necessarily destroying them.

appliance   Mechanical device used to support or align parts of the body to facilitate a particular function.

areolar tissue   Loose connective tissue.

arteriosclerosis   Hardening of the arteries.

arthrectomy   Removal of a joint by surgical means.

arthritis   Inflammation of a joint; there are many different types with different causes.

arthrodesis   Surgical fixation of a joint by fusion of the joint surfaces.

arthrography   X-ray visualization and recording of a joint by introduction of contrast medium into the joint for purposes of visualizing the joint structures.

arthropathy   Any joint disease.

arthroplasty   Reconstruction or plastic repair of a joint with the formation of a movable joint.

articulation   Place of union or junction between two or more bones of the skeleton.

aspiration   Withdrawal of fluid or gas from a cavity or joint space.

atherosclerosis   Fatty tissues in the blood vessels.

athlete's foot   Layman's term for fungal infection of the foot.

atrophy   Defect or wasting away or diminution in size of cells, tissues, or organs.

avulsion   The forcible or surgical removal of some part or all of a toenail.

balanced inlay   Flexible support worn in a shoe to balance weight and structure of the foot.

bars   Build-up on the exterior of the sole of a shoe to control distribution of weight to the foot.

Buerger's disease   Chronic, recurring inflammatory, vascular occlusive disease of the peripheral arteries and veins of the extremities.

bunion   Swelling of the outer side of the ball of the great toe, with a thickening of the overlaying skin and forcing of the toe toward the lesser toes.

bunionectomy   Removal of a bunion by arthroplasty of the first metatarsophalangeal joint.

bunionette   Bunion-like enlargement of the fifth metatarsal phalangeal joint of the little toe as a result of pressure over the lateral surface of the foot.

bursa   Sac or sac-like cavity filled with a fluid and situated in areas at which friction otherwise would develop.

bursitis   Inflammation of the bursa.

callosity   Circumscribed thickening of the skin; hypertrophy of the horny layer, from friction, pressure, or other irritations.

callus   Callosity; also used to describe the healing after the fracture of a bone.

cautery   Application of a burning agent (chemical or electrical), cold (as produced by carbon dioxide); actual cautery (as fire or actual burning), potential cautery (as by escharotic agent without applying heat).

cavum   A cavity or space.

cellulitis   Longstanding hardening and infection of cellular connective tissue.

chemosurgery   Surgical removal of diseased or unwanted tissue by application of caustic chemicals.

claudication   Pain in the calf during walking.

clavus molle   Soft corn found between the toes; also referred to as heloma molle.

clubfoot   Congenital deformity of the foot with multiple abnormalities.

collateral ligament   Ligament that connects one bone to another across joint spaces.

contracted toe   Also called hammertoe; toe bent upward at the middle joint.

corn   Horny induration and thickening of the skin (clavus), produced by friction and pressure and producing pain and irritation.

cryocautery   Destruction of tissue by application of extreme cold.

cyst   Pouch or sac, normal or abnormal, especially one that contains liquid or semisolid material.

debridement   Surgical removal of foreign material or devitalized tissue from an area.

dermatological   Having to do with skin.

dermatomycosis A superficial infection of the skin or its appendages by a fungus.

dermatophytosis (tinea pedis) Same as dermatomycosis but more often used specifically to designate infection of the skin of the feet.

diabetes A metabolic disorder that usually is caused by a faulty pancreas with the inability of the body to produce or properly utilize insulin, thereby producing high blood sugar with resulting sugar in the urine; condition usually is manifested in lower extremities in addition to elsewhere in body.

digiti flexus Flexed digits; hammertoes.

dorsalis pedis pulse Pulse on top of the foot.

dorsiflexion Backward bending or flexing, as of the hand or the foot.

eczema An inflammatory condition of the skin.

edema Swelling; the presence of an abnormally large amount of fluid in body tissues.

enthesopathy The result of an inflammatory process that involves the area where ligaments or tendons attach to bone (enthesis) by calcification or ossification (e.g., bone spur).

erythema Redness of the skin produced by congestion of the capillaries.

exostosis Bony growth projecting outward from the bone surface.

extensor Muscle or tendon on the dorsum of the foot that bends the foot or part of the foot up toward the leg.

Fabray's disease Inherited metabolic disease caused by a galactosidase deficiency.

fascia A sheet or band of fibrous tissue.

fibroma Tumor composed mainly of fibrous or fully developed connective tissues.

fissure Any crack, cleft, or groove, normal or otherwise, in skin of the foot, usually the heel.

flatfoot Flattening of the arch.

flexor Muscle that bends a limb or part (as opposed to an extensor).

functional insole   Lightweight, thin appliance to accommodate minor foot problems.

ganglion   Cyst of a joint capsule, tendon sheath, or aponeurosis.

gangrene   Local death of tissue.

gout   Hereditary metabolic diseased caused by hyperuricemia that is a form of acute arthritis and is marked by joint inflammation that usually begins in the great toe or the knee.

granulation tissue   Abnormal growth of vascular tissue associated with inflammation and healing.

hallux   The great toe, or first digit of the foot.

hallux valgus   Deviation of the first metatarsophalangeal joint, which causes the toe to drift laterally and the first metatarsal head to protrude medially.

Hansen's disease   *See* leprosy.

heloma   Corn of the foot.

hematoma   Localized collection of blood.

hemophilia   Hereditary blood disease marked by prolonged coagulation time and a failure of the blood to coagulate.

hydrotherapy   Use of water for therapeutic purposes.

hyperhidrosis   Excessive perspiration as a result of overactive sweat glands.

hyperkeratosis   Overgrowth of the horny layer of the epidermis.

hyperostosis   An abnormal growth of osseous tissue.

inflammation   Condition into which tissues enter as a reaction to injury or disease.

ingrown nail   Nail that breaks through the skin or tissue and causes pain.

keratotic   Any condition of the skin characterized by the formation of horny growths; excessive horny growth.

leprosy   Chronic communicable disease caused by microbacterium leprae, with neuropathy; sometimes called Hansen's disease.

lymphedema Abnormal accumulation of tissue fluid (lymph) in the interstitial spaces, causing swelling.

metatarsal One of the long bones of the foot.

metatarsalgia Pain and inflammation of the long bones of the foot.

Milroy's disease Chronic hereditary lymphedema of the legs.

Morton's syndrome Congenital short, hypertrophied second metatarsal bone with tenderness over the head of that bone.

mycotic Infection caused by fungus.

myofasciitis Inflammation of a muscle and its fascia.

myositis Inflammation of muscle tissue.

neoplasm A new growth of tissue (tumor) that serves no physiological function.

neuralgia Condition of pain along the course of a nerve.

neuritis Inflammation of a nerve.

neuroma A nerve tumor.

neurosyphilis Syphilis, a venereal or sexually transmitted disease that affects the neurological system; usually a syndrome of tertiary syphilis.

onychauxis Hypertrophy or thickening of the nail plate.

onychectomy Surgical removal of a nail.

onychia Inflammation with possible infection of nail bed and/or matrix that may result in the loss of the nail.

onycho Combining word form denoting relationship to the nails.

onychocryptosis Ingrown nail.

onychodysplasia Abnormal and exaggerated transverse curvature of the toe nails (pincer nails or incurvated toenails).

onychogryphosis Long-standing hypertrophy characterized by a curved or hooked nail (ram's horn nail); there is marked deformity and thickening, usually involving the longitudinal aspect of the nail with thickening and deformity.

onycholysis Loosening or detachment of nail from nail bed from the free edge of the toenail.

onychomadesis Loosening of the toenail from the posterior portion of the nail that may result in a complete loss of the nail.

onychomycosis A localized fungal infection of the nail or nail bed characterized by degeneration of the nail plate in which the nail becomes brittle, hypertrophic, and granular, with deformity and onycholysis.

onychopathy Any disease of the nails.

onychophosis Accumulation of the horny layers of the epidermis underlying the nail; clinically referred to as calloused nail grooves.

onychorrhexis Abnormal longitudinal striations of the nail plate with an associated brittleness and splitting of the nails.

orthodigita Correcting deformities of the toes and fingers.

orthomechanical therapy Treatment of foot and ankle problems with mechanical devices.

orthosis An orthopedic appliance or apparatus used to support, align, prevent, or correct deformities.

os Bone.

ossification Formation of bone; conversion of fibrous tissue or cartilage into bone.

osteoarthritis Chronic multiple degenerative joint disease.

osteochondritis Inflammation of both bone and cartilage.

osteoma Tumor of bone.

osteomyelitis Infection and inflammation of the bone.

osteotomy Surgical cutting of a bone.

palliative Affording relief but not a cure.

paronychia Infection, abscess, and inflammation of the nail bed, wall, and/or matrix.

pellagra A deficiency disease or syndrome caused by failure to absorb niacin.

pernicious anemia Destruction of red blood cells; chronic macrocytic anemia.

pes cavus Exaggerated height of long arch of the foot.

pes planus Deformed foot structure in which the bones of long arch have been altered to lower position.

pes valgo planus Deformed foot structure in which the bones of the long medial arch have been altered to a lower position with pronation and outward deviation and rotation of the foot.

phalangeal Phalanx (toe) bones.

phlebitis Inflammation of a vein.

plates Foot orthoses; rigid types used for correction, stabilization, and gait training of the foot.

podalgia Pain in the foot.

posterior tibial pulse Pulse in the foot located at the inside of the ankle.

pronation Result of a combination of factors in the tarsal and metatarsal areas of the foot that lowers the arch and allows the forefoot to splay, or turn outward, from the midline of the body.

pruritus Severe itching; may be a symptom of a disease process, such as an allergic reaction, or may be due to emotional factors.

psoriasis Chronic disease of the skin that consists of erythematous papules that coalesce to form plaques with distinct borders.

Raynaud's disease/syndrome Peripheral vascular disorder marked by abnormal vasoconstriction of the extremities on exposure to cold or emotional stress; most common onset occurs in women between 18 and 30 years of age.

reflex sympathetic dystrophy An excessive or abnormal response of the sympathetic nervous system after injury.

rheumatoid arthritis Chronic systemic disease marked by inflammatory changes in joints and related structures, generally thought to be caused by an autoimmune disease; results in crippling deformities.

sarcoidosis A chronic multisystem disease characterized by infiltration of the affected tissue and altered tissue architecture.

sesamoid   Small bone usually located beneath the head of the first metatarsal bone.

sprain   Joint injury whereby the supporting ligaments are stretched or ruptured but the continuity of the ligaments remains intact.

spur   Projecting body, as from a bone.

strain   Overstretching of the muscles as a result of excessive effort or undue exercise.

subluxation   Partial dislocation of a bone.

subungual   Beneath the nail.

syndactylism   Condition in which two or more digits are fused together; also referred to as web toes.

tailor's bunion   Bony overgrowth of the head of the fifth metatarsal with a medial deviation of the fifth toe.

tarsal bone   Of or pertaining to a bone in the tarsal region of the foot.

tarsal joint   Of or pertaining to the articulation between tarsal bones.

tarsus   The bones of the rear and midfoot, composed of seven bones called tarsal bones.

tendo-Achilles   Achilles tendon; the tendon that connects the posterior calf muscles to the heel bone; the thickest and strongest tendon in the body.

tendonitis   Inflammation of a tendon.

tenotomy   Surgical incision of a tendon.

tibialis anterior   A leg muscle that is attached to the foot and pulls the foot inward.

tinea pedis (athlete's foot)   An inflammatory reaction in the foot caused by fungal organisms (dermatophytosis).

tyloma   Callus of the foot.

ulcer   Open sore on the skin or mucous surface of a body organ, characterized by gradual disintegration and necrosis of tissues.

ungual   Pertaining to nails.

urticaria A vascular reaction of the skin characterized by a sudden general eruption of pale evanescent wheals or papules that are associated with severe itching.

valgus An eversion or turning out of the plantar aspect of the toes or the foot.

varicose Unnaturally swollen or enlarged and tortuous, as a vein, artery, or lymphatic vessel.

varus Inversion, or turning up, of the plantar aspect of toes or foot.

verruca Wart; tumorous growth of the skin caused by a virus.

xerosis Abnormal and excessive dryness of the skin with possible fissuring in older adults.

Comprehensive Podogeriatric Assessment and Chronic Disease Protocol

D eveloped under a contract from the Pennsylvania Department of Health, the Comprehensive Podogeriatric and Chronic Disease Assessment Protocol (Helfand Index) was developed by Temple University, School of Podiatric Medicine, in cooperation with the Pennsylvania Diabetes Academy; the Institute of Aging, Temple University; the Division of Endocrinology, Diabetes and Metabolic Diseases, Department of Medicine, Jefferson Medical College; and the Institute on Aging, University of Pennsylvania. The protocol includes a process to assess and evaluate common foot problems and to stratify at-risk patients. Once risks are identified and foot conditions are noted, a direction for care, education, and preventive measures can be prescribed.

The process collects information on the following:

- *History of present illness:* Includes primary foot problems and their relationship to ongoing health conditions and activities

- *Past history:* Includes the most common systemic diseases but needs to be augmented by primary and secondary risks as the evaluation evolves

- *Systems review and review of current medications:* Provides a cross-reference to potential risk diseases

- *Dermatological evaluation:* Focuses on multiple changes that affect pressure and mechanical keratosis, changes that occur in the toenail, infections, and preulcerative states

- *Foot orthopedic:* Highlights the most common foot deformities and syndromes in older adults and those with ongoing health conditions:

  —Arthritis

  —Hallux valgus (outward deviation of the great toe, commonly referred to as a bunion)

  —Anterior imbalance (inappropriate weight bearing; correlates with the plantar keratoma pattern noted later in the examination)

  —Digiti flexus (hammertoes and rotational deformities; correlates to imbalance, prominent metatarsal heads, and Morton's syndrome, which is an anatomic shortening of the first metatarsal segment that produces improper weight distribution and pressure areas)

  —Soft tissue inflammation

- *Vascular evaluation and risk stratification:* Identifies symptoms that are associated with arterial insufficiency and ischemia; *DP* refers to the dorsalis pedis pulse, and *PT* refers to the posterior tibial pulse; amputation, if present, is noted as above the knee (AKA), below the knee (BKA), forefoot (FF), and toes (T), which are particularly important in individuals with diabetes and arterial insufficiency

- *Neurological evaluation and risk stratification:* Identifies primary reflex and sensory changes

- *Footwear:* Information, assessment, and initial plan also are noted

- *Class finding:* Refers to what Medicare identifies as qualifiers for primary foot care for individuals with primary risk diseases (see in Tables 6, 7, and 8); note that all of the information listed in Table 8 should qualify in a similar manner in the future. The criteria for onychomycosis debridement coverage also are mandates of Medicare.

- *Classification of mechanical or pressure keratosis:* Modification of the program outlined by Merriman and Tollafield (1995)

- *Ulcer classification:* Adapted from Sims, Cavanagh, and Ulbrecht (1988) to provide an earlier identification of risk

- *Onychial grades at risk:* Modified and adapted from Strauss, Hart, and Winant (1998) to recognize earlier risk

- *Risk category—vascular:* Modified and adapted from Rutherford et al. (1997)

The final impression may not be a final diagnosis, but it identifies problems that require management, identifies latent risk factors and potential complications, provides a direction for education and prevention, and increases the awareness of foot health and care as an essential element for comprehensive patient care. It should be noted that foot care services for Medicare purposes must be provided by practitioners who are permitted by state license to render examination, diagnosis, and treatment of foot diseases (i.e., those with D.PM., M.D., or D.O. degrees).

Table 6. Primary Medicare risk diseases

Amyotrophic lateral sclerosis

Arteriosclerosis obliterans (arteriosclerosis of the extremities, occlusive peripheral arteriosclerosis)

Arteritis of the feet

Buerger's disease (thromboangiitis obliterans)

Chronic indurated cellulitis

Chronic thrombophlebitis[a]

Chronic venous insufficiency

Diabetes[a]

Intractable edema secondary to a specific disease (e.g., congestive heart failure, kidney disease, hypothyroidism)

Lymphedema secondary to a specific disease

Peripheral neuropathies involving the feet
  Alcoholism
  Associated with malnutrition and vitamin deficiency[a]
  Malabsorption (celiac disease, tropical sprue)
  Malnutrition (general, pellagra)

Peripheral vascular disease

Pernicious anemia
  Amyloid neuropathy
  Angiokeratoma corporis diffusum (Fabry's)
  Associated with carcinoma[a]
  Associated with diabetes[a]
  Associated with drugs and toxins[a]
  Associated with hereditary disorders
  Associated with leprosy or neurosyphilis
  Associated with multiple sclerosis[a]
  Associated with traumatic injury
  Associated with uremia (chronic renal disease)[a]
  Hereditary sensory radical neuropathy

Raynaud's disease

[a]Requires that the podiatric visit occur within 6 months of the patient having been seen by the attending or admitting long-term care physician who is treating the risk disease.

Table 7. Secondary risk diseases and conditions

Acromegaly	Hypertension
Alzheimer's disease	Mental illness
Ambulatory dysfunction	Mental retardation
Arthritis: degenerative joint disease	Paralysis
Arthritis: rheumatoid arthritis	Parkinson's disease
Cerebral palsy	Phlebitis
Cerebral vascular accident (stroke)	Poststroke
Chronic obstructive pulmonary disease	Posttrauma
Coagulation defect, anticoagulants	Preulcerative hyperkeratosis
Coagulation defect, hemophilia	Previous amputation: foot
Foot deformity	Previous amputation (toe)
Gout	Reflex sympathetic dystrophy
Hansen's disease	Sarcoidosis
Hemophilia	Sickle cell anemia
History of ulcer	Vascular insufficiency

Table 8. Tertiary risk conditions

Active chemotherapy
Anticoagulant therapy
Chronic steroid therapy
Heart valve replacement
Hemorrhagic disease
Immunosuppressive states
Joint implants
Renal failure, dialysis
Vascular grafts

Comprehensive Podogeriatric Assessment and Chronic Disease Protocol

Date of visit	MR#
Patient's name	
Date of birth	Age
Social security #	
Address	
City	State Zip code
Phone number	
Sex M F	Race B W A L NA
Weight (lbs.)	Height (in.)
Social status	M S W D Sep
Name of primary physician/health care facility	
Date of last visit	

History of present illness (check all that apply)

☐ Swelling of feet	☐ Painful feet
☐ Hyperkeratosis	☐ Onychial changes
☐ Bunions	☐ Painful toenails
☐ Infections	☐ Cold feet
☐ Other	
Quality	
Severity	
Duration	
Context	
Modifying factors	
Associated signs and symptoms	

Form development initiated by the Pennsylvania Department of Health.
This version appears in *Foot Health Training Guide for Long-Term Care Personnel* by Arthur E. Helfand; copyright © 2007 by Health Professions Press, Inc.

Comprehensive Podogeriatric Assessment and Chronic Disease Protocol (*continued*, page 2)

Past history (check all that apply)

	Diabetes mellitus:
☐ Heart disease	
☐ High blood pressure	☐ IDDM*
☐ Arthritis	☐ NIDDM*
☐ Circulatory disease*	☐ Hypercholesterol
☐ Thyroid	☐ Gout
☐ Allergy	☐ History: Smoking: OH
☐ Family-Social	

Systems review (check any problem areas)

☐ ENT	☐ Cardiovascular	☐ Genitourinary
☐ Eyes	☐ Musculoskeletal	☐ Neurological
☐ Skin/hair	☐ Endocrine	☐ Respiratory
☐ GYN	☐ Gastrointestinal	☐ Psychiatric
☐ Allergic	☐ Immunological	☐ Hematological
☐ Lymphatic		

Current medications:

Dermatological evaluation

☐ Hyperkeratosis*	☐ Xerosis
☐ Onychauxis (B2b)	☐ Tinea pedis
☐ Infection	☐ Verruca
☐ Ulceration*	☐ Hematoma
☐ Onychomycosis	☐ Rubor
☐ Onychodystrophy	☐ Preulcerative*
☐ Cyanosis* (BE)	☐ Discolored

Foot orthopedic

☐ Hallux valgus*	☐ Hallux rigidus-limitus*
☐ Anterior imbalance*	☐ Morton's syndrome*
☐ Digiti flexus*	☐ Bursitis
☐ Pes planus*	☐ Prominent met head*
☐ Pes valgo planus*	☐ Charcot joints*
☐ Pes cavus*	
☐ Other	

Form development initiated by the Pennsylvania Department of Health.
This version appears in *Foot Health Training Guide for Long-Term Care Personnel* by Arthur E. Helfand; copyright © 2007 by Health Professions Press, Inc.

Comprehensive Podogeriatric Assessment and Chronic Disease Protocol (*continued*, page 3)

Vascular evaluation

☐ Coldness* (C2)	☐ Claudication (C1)*
☐ Trophic changes* (B2a)	☐ Varicosities
☐ DP absent* (B3)	☐ Other
☐ PT absent* (B1)	☐ Amputation*
☐ Night cramps*	☐ AKA BKA FF T* (A1)
☐ Edema* (C3)	☐ Atrophy (B2d)

Risk category—vascular

0	☐ 0	No change
I	☐ 1	Mild claudication*
	☐ 2	Moderate claudication*
	☐ 3	Severe claudication*
II	☐ 4	Ischemic rest pain*
III	☐ 5	Minor tissue loss*
	☐ 6	Major tissue loss*

Neurological evaluation

☐ Achilles*	☐ Superficial plantar
☐ Vibratory*	☐ Joint position*
☐ Sharp/dull*	☐ Burning* (C5)
☐ Paresthesia* (C4)	☐ Other

Risk category—neurological

☐ 0 = No sensory loss

☐ 1 = Sensory loss*

☐ 2 = Sensory loss and foot deformity*

☐ 3 = Sensory loss, Hx ulceration, and deformity*

Items marked with an asterisk (*) denote Medicare qualifiers for **therapeutic shoes** for at-risk patients with diabetes and one or more of the following:

☐ History of partial or complete amputation of the foot

☐ History of previous foot ulceration

☐ History of preulcerative callus

☐ Peripheral neuropathy with evidence of callus formation

☐ Foot deformity

☐ Poor circulation

Form development initiated by the Pennsylvania Department of Health.
This version appears in *Foot Health Training Guide for Long-Term Care Personnel* by Arthur E. Helfand; copyright © 2007 by Health Professions Press, Inc.

Comprehensive Podogeriatric Assessment and Chronic Disease Protocol (*continued,* page 4)

Class findings (used as qualifiers for Medicare primary foot care coverage for patients with identified at-risk chronic diseases and/or conditions)	Onychomycosis (documentation of mycosis/dystrophy that is causing secondary infection and/or pain, which results or would result in marked limitation of ambulation)
A1 ☐ Nontraumatic amputation	☐ Discoloration ☐ Hypertrophy
B1 ☐ Absent posterior tibial	☐ Secondary infection ☐ Subungual debris
B2 ☐ Advanced trophic changes	☐ Limitation of ambulation ☐ Onycholysis and pain
B2a ☐ Hair growth (decrease or absent)	**Hyperkeratosis classification**
B2b ☐ Nail changes (thickening)	Grade 0 ☐ No lesion
B2c ☐ Pigmentary changes (discoloration)	Grade 1 ☐ No specific tyloma plaque but diffuse or pinch hyperkeratotic tissue present or in narrow bands
B2d ☐ Skin texture (thin, shiny)	
B2e ☐ Skin color (rubor or redness)	Grade 2 ☐ Circumscribed, punctate oval, or circular, well-defined thickening of keratinized tissue
B3 ☐ Absent dorsalis pedis	Grade 3 ☐ Heloma milliare or heloma durum with no associated tyloma
C1 ☐ Claudication	
C2 ☐ Temperature changes (cold)	Grade 4 ☐ Well-defined tyloma plaque with a definite heloma within the lesion, extravasation, maceration, and early breakdown of structures under the tyloma or callus layer
C3 ☐ Edema	
C4 ☐ Paresthesia	Grade 5 ☐ Complete breakdown of structure of hyperkeratotic tissue, epidermis, extending to superficial dermal involvement
C5 ☐ Burning	

Form development initiated by the Pennsylvania Department of Health.
This version appears in *Foot Health Training Guide for Long-Term Care Personnel* by Arthur E. Helfand; copyright © 2007 by Health Professions Press, Inc.

Comprehensive Podogeriatric Assessment and Chronic Disease Protocol (*continued*, page 5)

Plantar keratomata pattern

LT 5 4 3 2 1   RT 1 2 3 4 5

Ulcer classification

Grade 0 ☐ Absent skin lesions

Grade 1 ☐ Dense callus but not preulcer or ulcer

Grade 2 ☐ Preulcerative changes

Grade 3 ☐ Partial thickness (superficial ulcer)

Grade 4 ☐ Full-thickness (deep) ulcer but no involvement of tendon, bone, ligament, or joint

Grade 5 ☐ Full-thickness (deep) ulcer with involvement of tendon, bone, ligament, or joint

Grade 6 ☐ Localized infection (abscess or osteomyelitis)

Grade 7 ☐ Proximal spread of infection (ascending cellulitis or lymphadenopathy)

Grade 8 ☐ Gangrene of forefoot only

Grade 9 ☐ Gangrene of majority of foot

Onychial risk grades

Grade I ☐ Normal

Grade II ☐ Mild hypertrophy

Grade III ☐ Hypertrophic

☐ Dystrophic

☐ Onychauxis

☐ Mycotic

☐ Infected

☐ Onychodysplasia

Grade IV ☐ Hypertrophic

☐ Deformed

☐ Onychogryphosis

☐ Dystrophic

☐ Mycotic

☐ Infected

Form development initiated by the Pennsylvania Department of Health.
This version appears in *Foot Health Training Guide for Long-Term Care Personnel* by Arthur E. Helfand; copyright © 2007 by Health Professions Press, Inc.

Comprehensive Podogeriatric Assessment and Chronic Disease Protocol (*continued*, page 6)

Footwear satisfactory?	☐ yes ☐ no
Hygiene satisfactory?	☐ yes ☐ no
Stockings:	☐ nylon ☐ cotton ☐ wool ☐ other ☐ none
Assessment	

Clinical lab	
Imaging	
Prescription	
Services that are furnished for the evaluation and treatment of a patient who has diabetes with diabetic sensory neuropathy that results in a loss of protective sensation (LOPS) must include the following:	

Plan	
Podiatric referral	
Patient education	
Medical referral	
Special footwear	
Vascular studies	

1. A diagnosis of LOPS
2. A patient history
3. A physical examination that consists of findings regarding at least the following elements:
   a. Visual inspection of the forefoot, hindfoot, and toe web spaces
   b. Evaluation of protective sensation
   c. Evaluation of foot structure and biomechanics
   d. Evaluation of vascular status
   e. Evaluation of skin integrity
   f. Evaluation and recommendation of footwear
4. Patient education

Form development initiated by the Pennsylvania Department of Health.
This version appears in *Foot Health Training Guide for Long-Term Care Personnel* by Arthur E. Helfand; copyright © 2007 by Health Professions Press, Inc.

Index

Page numbers followed by *f* indicate figures; numbers followed by *t* indicate tables.